WALKING FOR FITNESS

About the Authors

LON H. SEIGER.   Dr. Seiger is a Professor of Health Education at Texas A & M University–Corpus Christi. An avid fitness walker for over twelve years, he has taught numerous college fitness walking classes and presented several fitness walking programs throughout the United States. Dr. Seiger is the lead author of seven books—four on walking and three on fitness and wellness.

Dr. Seiger holds a B.S. degree (Health and Physical Education) from Southeastern Oklahoma State University, an M.Ed. (Physical Education) from East Central Oklahoma State University, and an Ed.D. (Health Education) from Oklahoma State University. He is a Certified Health Education Specialist and a member of the American Alliance for Health, Physical Education, Recreation, and Dance and the American Association for Health Education.

JAMES L. HESSON.   Dr. Hesson is a professor in the Department of Biology and Biokinetics and the College of Applied Science and Technology at Black Hills State University in Spearfish, South Dakota. He has taught elementary, junior high, high school, and university. Dr. Hesson has been recognized for excellence in teaching and coaching.

Dr. Hesson earned his B.S. and M.S. degrees at the University of Nebraska–Lincoln. He earned his Ed.D. degree at Brigham Young University.

Dr. Hesson is the author of many articles as well as an author, coauthor, and contributing author of eighteen books. He is a member of the American College of Sports Medicine; the American Alliance for Health, Physical Education, Recreation, and Dance; the National Strength and Conditioning Association; Phi Delta Kappa; the Honor Society of Phi Kappa Phi; and the Human Anatomy and Physiology Society.

WALKING FOR FITNESS

Third Edition

Lon H. Seiger
Texas A&M University–Corpus Christi

James Hesson
Black Hills State University

Foreword by Charles F. Brock, Jr., M.D.

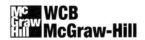

WCB McGraw-Hill

Boston, Massachusetts Burr Ridge, Illinois
Dubuque, Iowa Madison, Wisconsin New York, New York
San Francisco, California St. Louis, Missouri

WCB/McGraw-Hill

A Division of The **McGraw·Hill** Companies

WALKING FOR FITNESS:

Copyright © 1998, by The McGraw-Hill Companies, Inc. All rights reserved. Previous edition © 1994 by Brown & Benchmark Publishers, a Times Mirror Higher Education Group Inc., company. Printed in the United States of America. Except as permitted under the United States Copyright Act of 1976, no part of this publication may be reproduced or distributed in any form or by any means, or stored in a data base or retrieval system, without the prior written permission of the publisher.

 This book is printed on recycled, acid-free paper containing 10% postconsumer waste.

1 2 3 4 5 6 7 8 9 0 RRD/RRD 9 0 9 8 7

ISBN 0–697–34535–1

Publisher: *Ed Bartell*
Sponsoring editor: *Vicki Malinee*
Marketing manager: *Pamela S. Cooper*
Project manager: *Ann Morgan*
Production supervisor: *Deb Donner*
Designer: *K. Wayne Harms*
Cover designer: © *C. Chris Mooney/FPC International*
Art editor: *Joyce Watters*
Compositor: *Shepherd, Inc.*
Typeface: *10/12 Times Roman*
Printer: *R. R. Donnelley & Sons Company*

Library of Congress Cataloging-in-Publication Data

Seiger, Lon H.
    Walking for fitness/Lon H. Seiger, James Hesson; foreword by
Charles F. Brock, Jr.—3rd ed,
        p. cm.
    Includes bibliographical references (p. 183) and index.
    ISBN 0–697–34535–1
    1. Physical fitness.   2. Walking.   I. Hesson, James L.
II. Title.
GV502.S35   1998
613.7'176–dc21   97–20121
                                           CIP

www.mhhe.com

Dedication

To my wife Melissa and our three children, Von, Jensyn, and Keera; and to my Mom and Dad, sister Jodi, and brothers Radd and Darin—thanks for being "family."

Lon H. Seiger

To Margie, Jennifer, and David, for their patience, support, and love; to all my students, who have taught me how to help them learn; and to the greatest teacher of all, who is with us every step of the way in our walk through life.

James L. Hesson

CONTENTS

12

**Wellness Through Healthy
Lifestyles and Fitness   115**

Foreword

Medical research indicates that regular exercise performed at a moderate level of exertion can make a positive contribution to an individual's health. Exercise is especially beneficial for reducing the risk of cardiovascular disease and musculoskeletal conditions. For many, the emotional or psychological benefits of exercise are as important as the physical benefits. Most individuals report that they feel better once they begin a regular exercise program.

Walking is an attractive exercise alternative. It can be recommended for those who are healthy and can be prescribed for many who are not. Because walking is a familiar activity, it is relatively easy for the participant to commit to a walking program.

Cardiovascular disease and obesity are major health problems in the United States. Walking is an excellent exercise for those who are overweight because it reduces body fat and develops the cardiovascular system. In addition, the risk of injury is lower, since walking does not place as much stress on the bones and joints as some other popular activities do.

Walking for Fitness is a valuable source of information for those who desire a safe and enjoyable exercise program.

Charles F. Brock, Jr., M.D.

Preface

In 1989, *Walking for Fitness* was introduced as the first book on walking in the United States written exclusively for the college population. It is a text designed to educate and motivate you to adopt fitness walking and other positive behaviors for a healthy lifestyle.

Now in its third edition, *Walking for Fitness* has been developed to assist walkers of any age, sex, background, and skill level to acquire the knowledge, attitudes, and skills necessary for participation in a lifelong fitness walking program. Although designed primarily for an introductory course at the college level, the text can also be used in a variety of other settings. The material is presented in a style that is easy to understand for the beginning fitness walker, but intermediate and advanced levels of knowledge and skill can be achieved when the material is thoroughly mastered.

This text is not intended to be a total fitness book. The focus of *Walking for Fitness* is on the components of health-related physical fitness that are of greatest concern in our society—cardiovascular fitness and body composition.

Features

- The material is presented in a **reader-friendly style** that is **clear, concise,** and **practical.**
- **New photographs** have been added.
- The **figures** help complement the main ideas of the text.
- The **tables** offer easy-to-follow strategies to improve fitness and health.
- **Experiential activities** are found at the back of the book. The majority of these "hands-on" learning activities assess fitness and wellness behaviors. Other activities encourage participating in target behaviors to achieve a high level of fitness and wellness.
- A **helpful resource guide** is included for further information about fitness walking products, services, and tours.
- Included in the text is a **walking test, three walking programs,** and **guidelines for effective exercise.**

The first chapter provides a brief overview of the popularity of walking. Chapter 2 highlights the benefits for fitness walkers. Chapter 3 describes clothing and equipment. Chapter 4 details safety considerations. Guidelines for warm-up, cool-down, and flexibility are examined in chapter 5.

Chapter 6 describes the Rockport Fitness Walking Test. Chapter 7 illustrates fitness walking programs recommended by Rockport and the American Heart

Association. In addition, guidelines for effective exercise are presented for those who prefer to develop their own fitness walking program. Fitness walking techniques are presented in chapter 8.

The relationship of nutrition to wellness and guidelines for eating a healthy diet are examined in chapter 9. Key strategies for lifetime weight and fat control appear in chapter 10. Chapter 11 provides motivational strategies for sticking with a fitness walking program. Chapter 12 highlights the six interrelated components that make up a healthy lifestyle and strategies to attain a high level of well-being.

We believe you will enjoy reading *Walking for Fitness* and find the information important and useful. Each day of our lives we have conscious choices to make about our health. These choices have a cumulative effect and over time, will either enhance or detract from our present state of well-being. The target goal for this text is for you to choose fitness walking and other positive behaviors that can lead to a lifestyle of fitness and wellness. Since life is a journey, let us fully enjoy it. One way to do this is to value our health by taking positive action for it!

Acknowledgments

The authors wish to extend their appreciation to: Margie Hesson as a contributing author; David Baker for his outstanding photography; Jill Pankey and Lucia Vanderpool for their professional drawings; the models for their time and patience; and Dr. Bob Pankey, Dr. Robert Cox, Dr. Tito Guerrero, III, and Dr. Robert Furgason for their support.

General Information on Walking

Name of Sport: Walking

- Sport Description: Walkers must maintain unbroken contact with the ground. Thus, the rear foot must not leave the ground before the advancing foot has made contact. The leg must be momentarily straightened while a foot is on the ground.
- Forms: Striding, Fitness Walking, Racewalking, Hiking, Backpacking
- Average Time of Activity: 30–60 minutes
- Ease of Learning: Easy
- Equipment Costs to Get Started: $0–$100
- Regular Participation Costs: $0
- Lesson Costs: $0
- Schedule/Flexibility: High
- Injury Risk: Low
- Endurance Required: Aerobic (with oxygen)
- Strength Required: Low
- Skill/Coordination Required: Low
- Family/Social Activity: High
- Type: Individual
- Location: Land or Water
- Access to Facilities: Easy
- Ages: 1-year-old and up

The Walking Boom

Millions of Americans are now walking for the health of it!

Walking is easily the most popular form of exercise. Today, walking is riding a wave of popularity that draws its strength from a rediscovery of walking's flexibility, pleasures, and health-giving qualities. While other activities generate more conversation and media coverage, none of them approaches walking in number of participants. Approximately half of the 165 million adults in the United States claim they walk regularly. Each year the number is increasing.

While activities such as tennis, skiing, swimming, and others have gained great popularity over the years, walking has been widely practiced as a recreational and fitness activity throughout recorded history. For example, Presidents Lincoln, Jefferson, and Truman were avid walkers.

Walking is one of the safest and most effective forms of exercise to improve health, and develop and maintain physical fitness. Physicians, physical therapists, mental health counselors, and other medical professionals have long realized the value of walking for physical and psychological well-being.

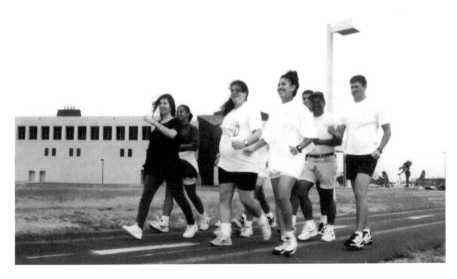

More and more Americans are walking to improve their health and fitness.

The Surgeon General's Report: Physical Activity and Health

This new report summarizes what has been discovered about physical activity and health. Among its major findings:

- people who are usually inactive can improve their health and well-being by becoming even moderately active on a regular basis.
- physical activity need not be strenuous to achieve health benefits.
- greater health benefits can be achieved by increasing the amount of physical activity through duration, frequency, or intensity.

The report also found that 60 percent of adults do not achieve the recommended amount of regular physical activity. In fact, 25 percent of all adults are not active at all. Inactivity, according to the Centers for Disease Control and Prevention, is comparable to smoking a pack of cigarettes a day. Other findings from this report are found in chapter 2.

The Surgeon General's Report should certainly encourage many people to become more active. Many of these new exercisers will choose walking as their exercise to become fit and shed the couch potato lifestyle—adding to the millions who are already walking.

The following section will define fitness walking and provide indicators that we are indeed experiencing a walking boom.

What Is Fitness Walking?

Fitness walking refers to the type of walking that produces health and fitness benefits. For you to be considered a fitness walker, you should walk briskly enough, long enough, and often enough to produce desirable health and fitness benefits. In addition, you should give proper attention to correct walking techniques, which will be discussed in chapter 8.

> **Refer to Activity 1a
> in the back of this book.**

Are There Walking Events?

There are over 10,000 walking events held every year, and this number is increasing. Volksmarching has become very popular. A volksmarch is a noncompetitive 6 mile (10 kilometer) walk that you can do with your class, a club, your family, your pet, or by yourself. Trails are selected for safety, scenic interest, historic areas, natural ability, and walkability and take about two hours to complete.

Voluntary health agencies such as the March of Dimes and the American Diabetes Association conduct annual walking events to raise money. Recently, promoters of many of the events that used to be for runners only are now encouraging walkers to enter. There has also been an increase in the number of race-walking events in our country. The Olympics have included the sport of racewalking since 1908.

Are There Walking Clubs?

Walking clubs are being formed all over the country. "The Walkers and Talkers" and "The Striders" are the names of two clubs that have turned fitness walking into an enjoyable social activity. There are now over 500 volksport clubs throughout the United States. Why not form a walking or volksport at your school or in your community? It's a healthy way to spend time with others and help host walking events.

Are Fitness Walking Courses Becoming Popular in Colleges and Universities?

There is a growing trend among colleges and universities to offer a walking class for credit. Over 100 institutions of higher learning now provide such a course. With the walking boom in high gear, experts predict classes in fitness walking will spread to most schools.

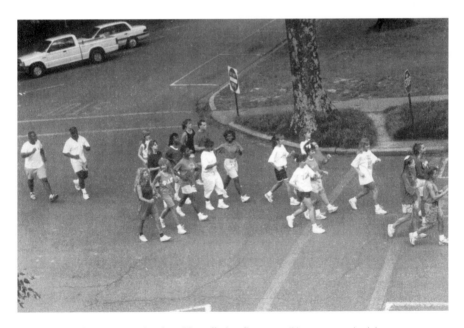

The number of colleges and universities offering fitness walking courses is rising.

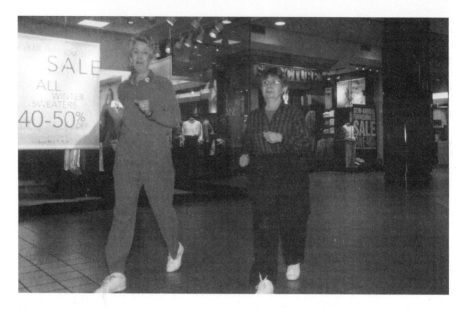

Mall walking has become popular as a safe, climate-controlled fitness activity.

What Is Mall Walking?

At many indoor shopping malls throughout the United States, walkers are allowed to exercise before the stores open or during normal hours of operation. This has provided many walkers with a comfortable and dependable place to exercise all year. Mall walking offers the additional attractions of personal safety and group participation.

Are There Fitness Walking Shoes?

The shoe industry provides further evidence of the growing popularity of fitness walking. Many years ago, it was difficult to find a good pair of walking shoes, but now most shoe companies make them. Some companies are including the design features of their fitness walking shoes in their dress shoes, so that it is now possible to wear comfortable shoes all day.

Where Can I Obtain Fitness Walking Information?

In recent years, there has been an increase in the amount of fitness walking information that is available. This information has appeared on the Internet, and in magazines, books, and brochures. It has also appeared on television, radio, videotape, and audiocassettes. Resources for fitness walking can be found in Appendix B.

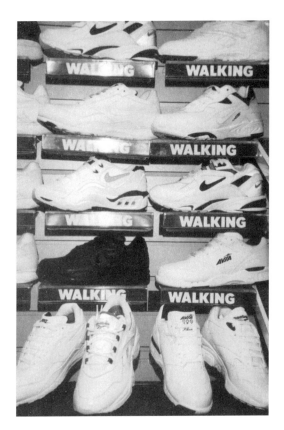

Numerous shoe companies now make walking shoes.

Are Walking Tours Available?

All over the world, walking tours are being promoted for walking enthusiasts. Numerous companies offer vacation packages in which two legs are better than four wheels. Walkers can experience the Swiss Alps, the rural footpaths of England, or they can view the wildlife, wildflowers, and spectacular scenery of the Rockies (see Appendix B).

Is Fitness Walking an Ideal Exercise?

In an age of high-tech exercise machines, why all of this interest in a form of exercise as old as the human race? There may be as many reasons for this interest as there are fitness walkers; however, when all reasons are considered, people are interested in fitness walking because it is an enjoyable and simple way to improve their health.

Fitness walking can be an escape from a high-tech lifestyle. There is no need for machines, videos, or expensive club memberships. You are not excluded from fitness

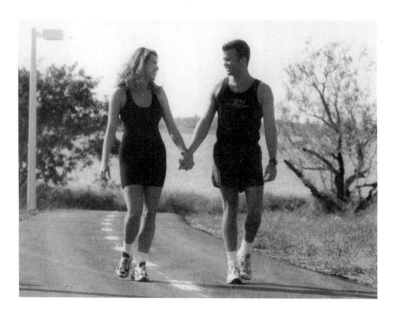

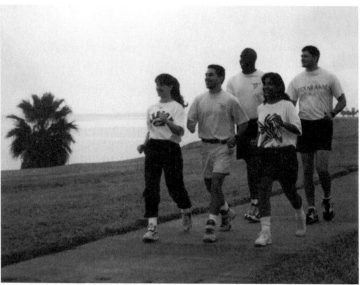

There are several types of walking to choose from: all the way from strolling to racewalking.

walking because of your age, body type, or skill level. Plus, walking is convenient—you can walk almost anywhere and at almost any time.

Fitness walking is a versatile exercise. The pace can be slow to start off and gradually increased as conditioning improves. The techniques are not difficult to learn, and there are several types of walking to choose from: strolling, everyday walking, hiking, backpacking, adventure walking, snowshoeing, stairwalking, fitness walking, and racewalking. You can probably think of other types, all of which allow you to find the best workout for your age, interest, and fitness level.

For these reasons and many others, health professionals are recommending fitness walking as an excellent form of exercise for all ages.

Can Walking Improve Physical Fitness?

For years, it was thought that walking would not provide enough exercise to produce any cardiovascular benefit; however, scientific research has now proven that fitness walkers are able to reach the exercise intensity necessary to improve cardiovascular fitness. When you use correct walking techniques and accelerated arm and leg movements, fitness walking involves most of the muscles in your body. Walking briskly increases the demand for oxygen, which makes your circulatory and respiratory systems work harder than usual, improving the functioning of your heart and lungs.

Is Walking Slow and Boring?

Of course not! Walking can be fast and interesting. Walking speeds may vary from a slow shuffle of less than 1 mile per hour to racewalking at speeds in excess of 10 miles per hour. World-class racewalkers can walk sub-6-minute miles and maintain that speed for more than 12 miles. Most people could not run one sub-6-minute mile, much less maintain that speed for 12 miles.

Fitness walkers generally walk a mile in about 12 to 17 minutes. Using proper form, with accelerated arm and leg swings, speed can be dramatically increased.

With a positive attitude, walking can be an exciting adventure. There are many entertaining things you can do while you walk. You could listen to a tape player to learn something new, listen to your favorite music, listen to the news, talk with friends and family, sing, solve personal problems, explore new areas, appreciate nature, pray, or meditate. Another suggestion for spicing up your walking routine is to play games. For example, count how many other walkers you see, remember all 50 states and their capitals, or go on a fantasy trip.

Is Walking Only for the Old and Injured?

It is true that fitness walking is an excellent exercise for older people, for cardiac patients, and for those who have been injured. However, fitness walking is a safe and effective form of exercise that is also being used by young, healthy individuals who want to become more fit.

Benefits of Fitness Walking

2

Why Exercise?

The leading causes of death in the United States are related to lifestyle (see table 2.1). One harmful lifestyle behavior is sedentary living. If you have an inactive lifestyle, there will be a decline in your body's ability to function. If you allow this deterioration to continue, eventually one of your organ systems will not be able to perform its life-sustaining function. When this occurs, you will experience a life-threatening illness or death.

Long before death, however, there may be years of "not feeling very well"— nothing definite, no specific symptoms. The feeling that life is difficult rather than enjoyable, that it is all you can do to plow through another day—these are feelings frequently expressed by people in poor physical condition.

The good news is that a moderate amount of exercise on a regular basis will improve the functioning of your body. Exercise can help you look better, feel better, and enjoy life.

Why Aerobic Exercise?

You are an aerobic organism. The term *aerobic* (a-rō'-bik) describes life forms that require oxygen. You could live weeks without food, days without water, but only minutes without oxygen. How well your body operates depends on your ability to get oxygen to every living cell.

Oxygen is brought into your body with the air you breathe into your lungs. Approximately one-fifth of normal, unpolluted air is oxygen. Some of the oxygen that enters your lungs is transferred into your blood. Your heart then pumps the oxygenated blood to all of your cells.

Any life-style behavior that reduces the functioning of your respiratory or circulatory system reduces your ability to get life-sustaining oxygen to your cells. Sedentary living reduces your ability to deliver oxygen to all parts of your body. This decline in oxygen delivery could be considered a slow form of suffocation and results in "not feeling very well."

If this deterioration continues, eventually you will only be able to take in enough oxygen to sustain your life in a resting state. This does not leave any room for adjustment to an increased demand, such as a physical or an emotional emergency. A poorly conditioned person may experience a sudden demand for increased oxygen delivery. Since his or her body is not capable of delivering more oxygen to the heart

Table 2.1 Deaths and Death Rates for the 10 Leading Causes of Death, Preliminary Data for 12 Months Ending with June 1996

Rank	Cause of Death	Number	Death Rate (per 100,000 people)
	All causes	2,321,995	879.0
1.	Disease of the heart	736,844	278.9
2.	Malignant neoplasms (Cancer)	541,123	204.8
3.	Cerebrovascular diseases (Strokes)	159,820	60.5
4.	Chronic obstructive pulmonary disease	103,553	39.2
5.	Accidents and adverse effects	93,990	35.6
	Motor vehicle accidents	43,764	16.6
	All other accidents and adverse effects	50,227	19.0
6.	Pneumonia and influenza	82,875	31.4
7.	Diabetes mellitus	60,249	22.8
8.	Human immunodeficiency virus infection	39,978	15.1
9.	Suicide	30,348	11.5
10.	Chronic liver disease and cirrhosis	25,387	9.8
	All other causes	447,847	169.5

Source: *Monthly Vital Statistics Report, Vol. 45, No. 13,* April 30, 1997. U.S. Department of Health and Human Services, National Center for Health Statistics.

muscle, which is now working harder than normal, some of the oxygen-starved heart muscle tissue may die. The affected tissue can no longer contract; therefore, the heart may not be able to continue to pump oxygenated blood to any of the other living cells of the body. This is a simplified explanation of one type of heart attack. Of course, without a continuous supply of life-sustaining oxygen, the other cells of the body cannot survive.

Since you are an aerobic organism, exercises that improve your ability to obtain and use oxygen (aerobic exercises) are beneficial. They stimulate the development of your oxygen delivery system. Aerobic exercises typically use large muscle groups in a rhythmic and continuous manner. Listed in table 2.2 are some of the benefits of aerobic exercise.

Why Fitness Walking?

Fitness walking is an excellent aerobic exercise for many reasons.

Lifetime Exercise

To get the greatest benefit from exercise, it must be consistent and lifelong, 12 months a year, every year. Because it is a low-impact activity, walking can be enjoyed by people of all ages.

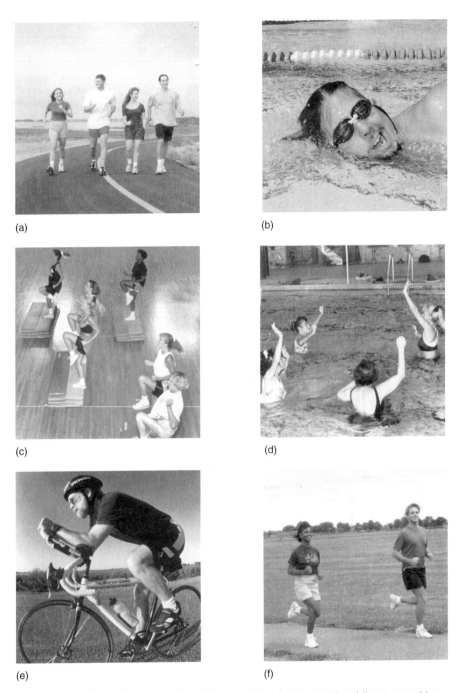

Six major aerobic activities: (a) walking, (b) swimming, (c) step aerobics, (d) water aerobics, (e) bicycling, and (f) jogging.

Table 2.2 Benefits of Aerobic Exercise

The following benefits have been reported as a result of a moderate amount of aerobic exercise performed on a regular basis. All of these benefits are still under investigation. Some have been studied more thoroughly than others. Biological adaptation to exercise is a gradual process that requires consistent and long-term participation.

Heart
—Increased strength of the heart muscle
—Increased stroke volume
—Increased cardiac output
—Increased heart volume
—Decreased resting heart rate
—Decreased exercise heart rate at a standard workload
—Decreased risk of cardiovascular disease
—Decreased risk of heart attack
—Decreased severity of heart attack if one does occur
—Increased chance of surviving a heart attack if one does occur

Blood
—Increased blood flow
—Increased total blood volume
—Increased number of red blood cells
—Increased oxygen-carrying capacity of the blood
—Increased high-density lipoproteins (HDL)
—Increased ability to extract oxygen from the blood
—Decreased harmful blood fats
—Decreased total cholesterol

Blood Vessels
—Increased size of capillaries
—Increased number of open capillaries
—Increased peripheral circulation
—Increased coronary circulation
—Decreased resting blood pressure for some individuals
—Decreased risk of atherosclerosis

Lungs
—Increased minute volume of air
—Increased rate of breathing during exercise
—Increased volume per breath during exercise

Body Fat
—Decreased total body fat
—Decreased percent body fat
—Maintenance of healthy body-fat level
—Decreased appetite if exercise is performed just before a meal
—Decreased total body weight

Table 2.2 (continued)

Muscle
—Increased lean body weight
—Increased muscle tissue
—Increased muscle strength
—Increased muscle endurance

Bone
—Increased bone density
—Increased bone and joint strength
—Decreased risk of osteoporosis

Connective Tissue
—Increased tendon, ligament, and joint strength

Endurance
—Increased work efficiency
—Increased sports performance
—Increased ability to use oxygen
—Increased physical ability to meet emergency situations
—Increased recovery after hard work
—Increased cardiovascular endurance
—Increased functioning of oxygen supply organ systems

Resistance to Disease
—Increased resistance
—Increased health

Appearance
—Improved appearance
—Improved posture
—Decreased waistline

Stress
—Decreased emotional stress

Psychological
—Increased self-concept
—Increased positive attitude, positive feeling
—Increased self-confidence
—Increased self-discipline
—Increased independence for many older citizens
—Decreased depression
—Increased soundness of sleep
—Decreased mental tension
—Increased social interaction with healthy people
—Increased resistance to fatigue
—Increased feeling of success
—Increased enjoyment of leisure time
—Increased enjoyment of work
—Increased quality of life, sense of well-being

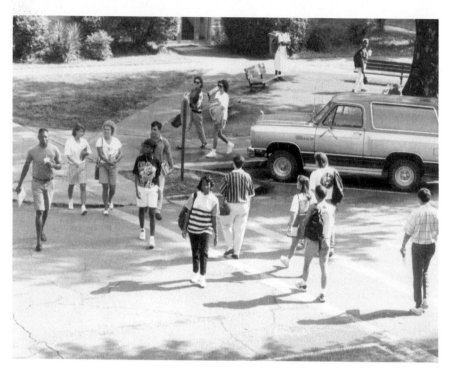

Walking is a convenient and enjoyable method of transportation.

Almost Everyone Can Participate

Walking has few restrictions. Almost everyone can participate in fitness walking. No special sports skills are necessary in order to achieve a beneficial amount of exercise.

If you are overweight, walking is ideal because it puts less strain on your bones and joints than some of the other aerobic activities.

Natural and Safe Exercise

Walking is one of the most natural exercises for the human body. Your body was designed for movement, not inactivity.

Walking is also a safe exercise. Many former joggers have converted to fitness walking. The force of landing on each foot during jogging is about three and one-half to four times your body weight. In contrast, the force of landing on each foot during walking is about one to one and one-half times your body weight. Therefore, joint and muscle injuries are less likely to occur with a walking program.

Inexpensive

Fitness walking does not require expensive facilities, equipment, or membership. The most expensive and important equipment for fitness walking is a good pair of walking shoes. However, such shoes can be worn in a variety of situations and over

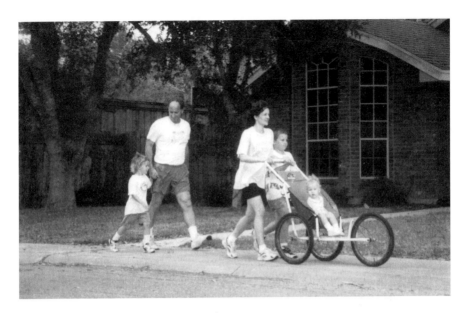

Family and friends can enjoy walking together.

a long period of time. Therefore, considering the cost per hour of use, walking shoes are less expensive than most other exercise equipment.

Of course, as fitness walking continues its rapid growth in popularity, creative people will develop innovative products, facilities, clothing, equipment, and memberships that will find a market. If you enjoy these new products and services, have a desire for them, and can afford them, that's fine—but remember that they are not necessary for you to gain the benefits from fitness walking.

Weight Loss

Seventy-four percent of Americans 25 or older are overweight according to a 1996 Harris Poll report. Fitness walking is an excellent way to lose weight. Since so many people are interested in losing excess body fat, chapter 10 in this book is devoted to this important benefit of fitness walking.

Easier to Start and Stick With

Walking is a familiar activity, one in which you already have some skill. Since you know how to do it and can do it almost anywhere, it is relatively easy to start a walking exercise program.

The dropout rate for fitness walking is lower than for other exercise programs. Walking is convenient and accessible, and it can be used as a form of transportation. Walking can be combined with other enjoyable activities, such as sightseeing and carrying on a conversation. Because walking is more enjoyable than some of the other fitness activities, you are more likely to stick with your exercise program.

Posture

Fitness walking promotes good posture by strengthening many of your muscles. Good posture allows you to function more effectively, expending a minimum amount of energy. With good posture, there is less strain on your muscles, tendons, ligaments, and joints. Good posture also conveys an impression of alertness, confidence, and attractiveness.

Social Activity

Walking is an excellent family and group activity. It can be a social activity and a fitness activity at the same time. Whereas joggers often have difficulty maintaining a conversation while they exercise, walkers are likely to maintain a conversation due to the lower intensity and longer duration of many walking programs.

Walking provides an excellent opportunity for family members and friends to spend regular time together. It provides a time to discuss personal and family needs, wants, goals, and dreams. Instead of going out for dinner, dessert, or a drink, why not go out for a walk together?

Get Fit for Sports

You can start slowly with fitness walking and gradually build to a high level of fitness. For people who have not been exercising, walking is recommended as a starter program to prepare for participation in sports.

Rehabilitation of Injuries

Walking can be an excellent exercise to help an individual recover from injuries, especially leg injuries. When muscles are not used, they atrophy (decrease in size and strength). Walking can be an important exercise in the recovery process because the intensity of the exercise and the workload placed on the injured tissue can be controlled to a greater extent than in many other exercises. Walking helps rebuild or maintain muscle tissue as the injury heals.

Cardiac Rehabilitation

Walking is the primary exercise in many cardiac rehabilitation programs. It is a good exercise for those recovering from heart attacks because walking is an exercise that they

- are familiar with,
- are not afraid of,
- can continue for the rest of their lives,
- can easily monitor,
- can start at a low level, and
- can progressively increase.

Walking gets heart attack victims on their feet again. It helps them regain some control of their lives and feel optimistic about the future.

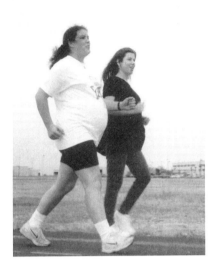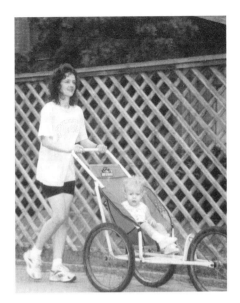

Walking is an excellent exercise during and after pregnancy.

Exercise during Pregnancy

Walking is one of the safest and best exercises during pregnancy. Many women, when they find out they are pregnant, stop all physical activity and become totally deconditioned, ironically for the most demanding physical activity of their lives. When they do finally give birth, they are in their weakest physical condition as a result of nine months of deconditioning. Adequate exercise and good nutrition bring many benefits to the developing child as well as to the mother.

Fitness walking is a good exercise for pregnant women because it is a low-impact activity. Also, the intensity level can be easily monitored and adjusted to the fairly rapid biological changes that occur during pregnancy.

Exercise after Pregnancy

Walking is an excellent exercise after pregnancy. A new mother can start slowly and progress gradually as her fitness level improves. She can begin immediately to lose excess body fat she may have gained during pregnancy and begin to get her figure back. Walking after pregnancy also promotes cardiovascular endurance—an important attribute for a new parent.

Walking is not only a good exercise, it is also good for stress management. It provides an opportunity to enjoy being outdoors. A new mother can take her baby along in a stroller; the stimulation of new surroundings is good for young children. She might choose to leave the baby with another caregiver for 30 to 60 minutes while taking an exercise break.

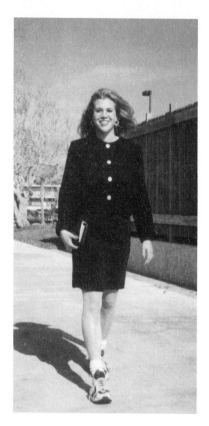 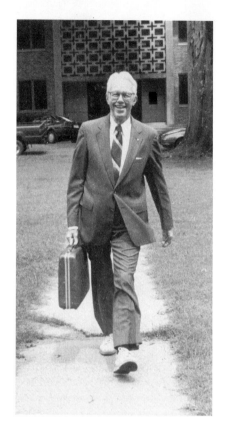

Walking can fit into anyone's daily routine.

Fits in with Your Daily Routine

You can choose to walk at a time that best fits your schedule. Some people prefer to walk early in the morning to start the day. Others prefer to walk late at night. Still others choose to walk at noon or during breaks. These are only a few of the ways people fit walking into their daily routine.

> **Refer to Activity 2a
> in the back of this book.**

Psychological Benefits

Regular fitness walkers have come to appreciate the value of this exercise for their psychological well-being. In fact, many walkers report that the psychological benefits from walking are just as important, if not more important, than the physical benefits. Figure 2.1 highlights some of the major psychological benefits from a regular program of fitness walking.

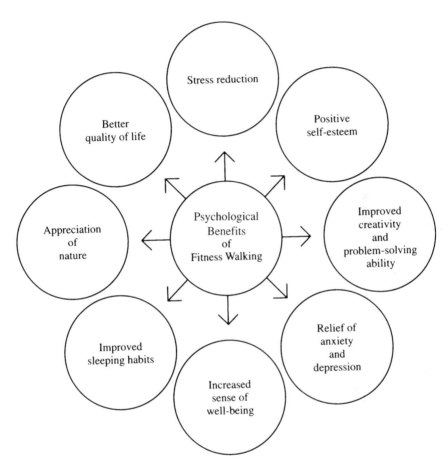

Figure 2.1
The Psychological Benefits of Fitness Walking

Clothing and Equipment

3

One of the advantages of fitness walking is that you don't need to spend a lot of money on special clothing and equipment. Some activities, such as skiing and scuba diving, require expensive equipment that might be used only once or twice a year. Most fitness walking clothing and equipment is relatively inexpensive and can be used every day.

The most important piece of clothing or equipment you can buy for fitness walking is a good pair of walking shoes. They may seem expensive when you first look at the selling price; however, if you take the time to calculate the cost per hour of use and the value of your health, you will find high-quality walking shoes to be a good investment.

Walking Shoes

Approximately 87 percent of all Americans have suffered from foot problems. Many are caused by wearing shoes that do not fit properly or shoes that are worn out. When shopping for shoes, it is wise to spend a little extra time and money to get good quality and a proper fit.

When shopping for fitness walking shoes, be sure to allow enough time. Do not try to do it in five minutes. Be a good comparison shopper. Try on at least three different brands and as many styles as possible. Even if a shoe is ranked as the best, or the most popular, it may not fit you as comfortably as another brand or model.

When you try on walking shoes, test them on a hard surface instead of the padded carpet that is commonly found in shoe stores. This test will help you determine the amount of cushion and comfort the shoes provide.

Outer Sole

The outer sole is the material on the bottom of a shoe. It should be made from a durable material. A good walking shoe has a rocker-shaped sole, which helps your foot rock forward from heel to toe. Walking shoes have a tread design for traction; however, it is not as deep as commonly found on running shoes.

Some people experience eversion when they walk or run. Eversion is the anatomical term for a movement in which the bottom of the foot turns outward. Commercially, the term *pronation* is being used instead of eversion to describe this foot movement and has gained popular acceptance. A shoe with antipronation construction is designed to keep the sole of your foot from turning too far outward. If

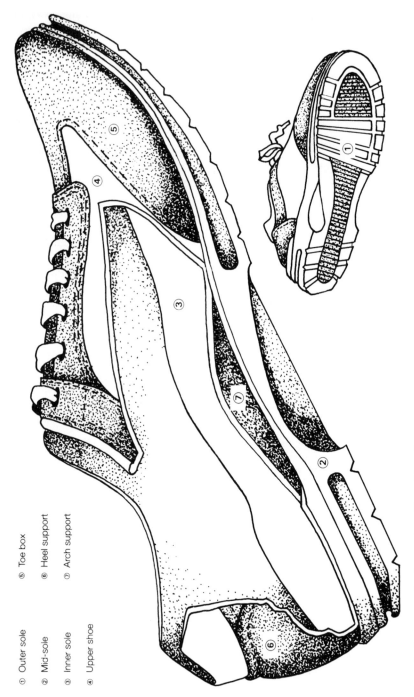

① Outer sole   ⑤ Toe box

② Mid-sole   ⑥ Heel support

③ Inner sole   ⑦ Arch support

④ Upper shoe

Important components of a good quality walking shoe.

excessive pronation occurs with every step, extensive jogging or walking could eventually result in injury. Therefore, some of the better running and walking shoes have antipronation construction for those who need the extra support.

Mid-Sole

The mid-sole is a cushioning layer between the outer and inner soles. Since the primary purpose of the mid-sole is to absorb shock, it can be made from a variety of materials and designed in many different ways.

There is no exact way for most people to determine when the mid-sole has lost its ability to absorb shock. The outer sole and upper part of the shoe may look fine, but, if the mid-sole has lost its resiliency, it is time to get a new pair of walking shoes.

Inner Sole

The inner sole makes direct contact with the foot. This sole should include an arch support and a heel cup. Some shoes have an arch support that can be added to, or removed from, the inner sole. The inner sole may also provide additional air or gel cushioning.

The inner sole can be removed from many walking shoes. One advantage of this is to let the inner sole air out after a workout. A second advantage is that it can be replaced if it wears out. A third advantage is that a podiatrist or an orthopedic doctor can make an inner sole that is just right for your foot.

Upper Shoe

The upper shoe is often made of leather because it is a durable, supple material. The toe box portion of the shoe should be wide enough so that the front part of your foot can spread out. This will allow you to push off with all of your toes.

The heel of the upper shoe should include a stiff material to provide support and to hold your foot in position. Good walking shoes often have a notch at the top of the heel support to minimize irritation of the Achilles tendon.

Some walking shoes also have reflective material as a safety measure for those who walk in the dark.

Size and Comfort

Try on both shoes. One of your feet may be longer than the other. Purchase shoes that are comfortable for the longest foot. You may need to wear an extra sock on the smaller foot if there is a big difference.

You may find that different brands of shoes fit differently, even if the sizes marked on the shoes are the same. Also, the size of your feet may have changed since your last shoe purchase. If you choose to buy your walking shoes through a mail order company, make sure it has a good return policy.

Walking shoes should not require a "break in" period. However, it is still a good idea to alternate your old shoes with your new shoes for a couple weeks. This allows your feet to adjust to the change gradually.

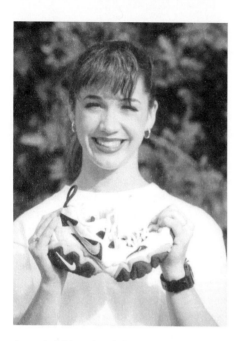

A good walking shoe is flexible.

Walking shoes should fit comfortably, not too tight or too loose. They need to be long enough and wide enough. Fitness walking shoes should be at least one-fourth of an inch longer than your big toe, and your feet should not feel squeezed into a shoe that is too narrow. Do not sacrifice comfort for name brand, style, or sale price. It is important that your walking shoes be comfortable.

Flexibility

All three soles and the upper shoe should bend at the ball of your foot. A good walking shoe should not be stiff at this point.

Weight

Racewalking shoes are lighter than training shoes. A few ounces of additional weight may make a difference in a race. However, most fitness walkers prefer training shoes that are more durable.

Quality

Look carefully at walking shoes. Is the shoe made from quality materials? Is it put together well? Is the stitching done carefully? Is the upper shoe securely fastened to the mid-sole?

Fitness walking shoes are an investment in your health. Invest wisely; insist on quality.

Shopping Guide

Brad Ketchum, Jr. and Tom Brunick offered the following tips for selecting walking shoes in *Walking* magazine.

1. **Toe box.** The most important thing a walker needs in a shoe is a good fit, and fit begins with the toe box. Look for a rounded, roomy toe compartment with three-dimensional space—shoes that taper or recede toward the toes might literally cramp your (walking) style. There's no need to sacrifice fit for fashion.

2. **Lacing.** A good lacing system can customize the fit of a walking shoe. Almost all models now come with variable-width or dual lacing, which includes at least one set of double eyelets near the top of the shoe. Walkers with narrow feet should use the outer eyelets to pull the upper tight; those with wide feet can use the inner eyelets for more room. Among the latest lacing features are plastic straps and stretch panels to further perfect the fit.

3. **Interiors.** Look for three features inside a walking shoe: a padded heel collar to reduce chafing, a padded tongue to protect the forefoot, and a smooth, absorbent lining. Also check the inner sole. As previously mentioned, most are removable so that they can be aired out or replaced.

4. **Heel cup.** The heel cup provides support in a walking shoe. Most shoes have plastic heel cups sewn inside the upper. Many also have smaller, external "stabilizers," which create a stable platform to keep your heel from rolling from side to side. For even more support, look for a heel cup that extends all the way around the side of the shoe toward the arch.

5. **Rocker profile.** Look for a natural, heel-to-toe curve. When the shoe is placed on a table, neither the heel nor the toe should touch the surface. Models with extreme rocker bottoms will rest on the middle of their outer soles. The heel should also be slightly beveled for proper heel strike.

Some walkers prefer to have two pairs of walking shoes. Switching between two pairs of shoes gives your feet a break from wearing only one pair. Also, if the shoes get wet, they will have time to dry between workouts.

**Refer to Activity 3a
in the back of this book.**

Clothing

Clothing for fitness walking should be comfortable, allow for freedom of movement, and make you feel good about your appearance. Cotton socks are excellent for absorbing moisture. For extra comfort, you may want to wear two pairs. Another option would be to buy socks that have extra cushioning in the heel and forefoot

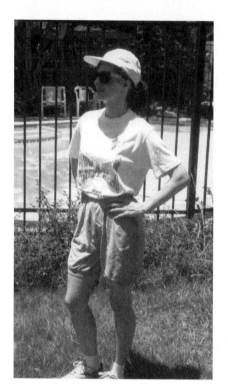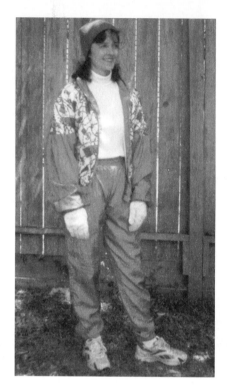

Hot and cold weather clothing.

area. This extra cushioning may reduce friction and help prevent blisters. A sports bra for women, and an athletic supporter for men, provide firm support and generally make fitness walking more comfortable.

Hot Weather Clothing

Light-colored and loose-fitting clothes are cooler than dark, tight clothes during hot weather. Light-colored clothing reflects some of the sun's rays, and loose-fitting clothing allows air to circulate next to your skin.

Walking shorts should allow free and easy movement. Light-weight shorts with built-in briefs add support with little increase in bulk. Shorts that are made of thick material might have a bulky inseam that could rub on the inside of your thighs. Another advantage of light-weight shorts is that they dry quickly. It is possible to rinse them out after each workout and have them clean and dry for the next day.

Shirts that are loose fitting and made of natural fabrics, such as cotton, absorb perspiration and allow air next to your skin.

A good hot-weather walking hat should have a raised crown with vents to allow air to circulate between the top of the hat and your head. In sunny weather, the brim of the hat should protect your eyes and forehead from the harmful rays of the sun. On hot, sunny days a hat helps prevent headaches and fatigue.

Cold Weather Clothing

For fitness walking in cold weather, dress in layers of clothing. This will allow you to remove layers to regulate your body temperature as you walk. Keeping warm while exercising in cold weather is not as much of a problem as you might think. Approximately 75 percent of the energy released during muscle contraction is heat energy; therefore, your muscles produce a lot of heat during exercise. You can use your layers of clothing to control how much heat you want next to your skin.

The first layer of clothing next to your skin should be made of a material that will keep you warm and dry. It should draw moisture away from your skin; it is difficult to stay warm if you are wet. This layer should be a loose-weave fabric with air spaces that can hold warm air next to your skin.

The next layer on your upper body might be a long-sleeved t-shirt or a turtleneck. On top of that, add a wool pullover or a sweatshirt.

The top layer could be a cotton sweatsuit or a garment made of a synthetic fabric, depending on the weather conditions. If the weather is wet, the outer layer should be waterproof. If the weather is cold and windy, the outer layer should serve as a windbreaker.

Warm-up suits with air vents enhance evaporation, thus reducing the moisture content inside the suit. These warm-up suits hold most of the heat in while allowing the moisture to escape.

A knit hat is recommended for cold weather. Wool is popular. A hat or hood helps hold in body heat. As much as two-thirds of your body heat can be lost from your head if it is not covered.

Gloves or mittens should be worn during fitness walking because the fingers are especially vulnerable to the cold. A woven material allows perspiration to be drawn away from your skin, whereas a solid synthetic material allows perspiration to accumulate. Natural fabrics, such as cotton or wool, work well.

Body Suits

Body suits are available that are made of lycra or lycra blend material. They conform to the shape of your body like a layer of skin. If a body suit is comfortable, if it does not restrict your movement, and if you feel good in it, this may be a good choice of walking clothing for you.

Sauna Suits

Rubber suits or sauna suits are dangerous and should not be worn. These suits are made of nonporous material; air and moisture cannot pass through. Sauna suits have elastic at the neck, wrists, waist, and ankles; during exercise, the air between the suit and your skin becomes hot and humid. It is possible to experience extreme heat and humidity inside a sauna suit, even on a comfortable day; thus, heat cramps, heat exhaustion, and heat stroke can occur.

Some people wear sauna suits during exercise so they will sweat more. Heavy sweating may result in a rapid but temporary weight loss. However, the pounds lost are due to fluid loss, not fat loss. The fluid and weight are quickly regained with any food or liquid intake. This is an unhealthy and ineffective way to attempt to lose weight. A healthy way to lose weight and body fat is to use more calories than you consume over a period of time.

Equipment

Fitness walking equipment can make walking safe and enjoyable.

Sunglasses

Sunglasses are important to protect your eyes from the harmful direct rays of the sun and from reflected glare. The best sunglasses to use are the ones that provide UV (ultraviolet) protection. As a fitness walker, it is possible to experience dizziness and temporary vision impairment if your eyes are not shielded from direct sunlight.

Reflective Material

Some people walk when it is dark. This is especially true during the winter months, when the daylight hours are short. You can put reflective tape on your walking clothes and shoes, and reflective vests are available. If you decide not to use reflective material, at least wear light-colored clothing that can be seen more easily at night.

Pulsemeter

A pulsemeter allows you to monitor your heart rate while you are walking. You need to reach a prescribed exercise heart rate to receive an adequate cardiovascular training effect. A pulsemeter can inform you when you have reached your exercise heart rate. It provides feedback that can be used to stay at the correct exercise heart rate for the duration of your walk.

Pedometer

A pedometer is a device that measures how far you walk. This is usually done by counting the number of steps you take. On some models, you need to pre-set your approximate stride length.

Backpack and Fanny Packs

Backpacks are useful for one-day hikes and weekend trips. In your backpack, you can carry first aid items, a change of socks, and extra layers of clothing. Waist packs, or fanny packs, are also available to carry small items, such as keys, during your workout.

Hand Weights

Hand weights may be carried during fitness walking to increase your muscular effort, energy expenditure, oxygen demand, and heart rate. Beginners should not carry weights. The additional exercise load could be harmful for an unconditioned beginner. Hand weights should only be considered by intermediate or advanced fitness walkers.

Walking Sticks and Canes

Some people use walking sticks and canes when walking. They can serve as a tool to ward off aggressive animals and human beings. A walking stick and a cane differ in that any stick can be a walking stick but a walking cane must bear weight safely, have a comfortable handle, and have a rubber tip.

Safety

4

Medical Clearance

Fitness walking has many benefits; however, as with any activity that involves human movement, care must be taken to avoid injury. You should get medical clearance from your physician before starting a fitness walking program. Also, knowing some of the possible dangers in advance will enable you to walk safely.

```
Refer to Activity 4a
in the back of this book.
```

Listen to Your Body

Too much exercise the first day can result in unnecessary pain and injury. When you begin an exercise program, start slowly.

Some mild muscle soreness a day or two after beginning a new exercise program is common, and can be relieved with static stretching and aerobic exercise. Both of these should be included in your fitness walking workouts.

If you progress slowly into your new exercise program, you should not experience any extreme pain. Pain is generally an indication of injury. If you do experience extreme pain, you should stop exercising and seek medical attention. Learn to listen to your body for feedback about the effects of your fitness walking program. Fitness walking should feel good, and you should look forward to your next session.

Walking during Extreme Weather Conditions

One excuse many people use for not exercising on a regular basis is the weather. Although there is a wide range of weather conditions in which fitness walking can be performed, there are also some dangers of exercising in extreme weather conditions. If you know the dangers and take precautions, the weather should rarely be an excuse for not exercising.

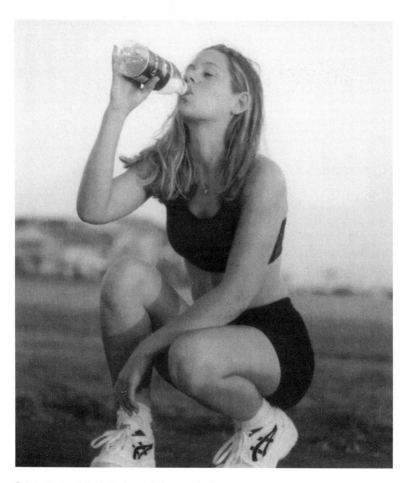

Drink plenty of fluids before, during, and after exercise.

Hot Weather Walking

The dangers of exercising in hot weather should be taken seriously. A loss of body fluid can impair performance, and an excessive loss can lead to heat cramps, heat exhaustion, or heat stroke. Those who are poorly conditioned, overfat, older, and not acclimatized to exercise in the heat have a higher risk. People who have previously suffered from heat disorders should be especially careful.

To reduce the risk of developing heat disorders, drink plenty of water about 30 minutes before walking. Continue to drink small amounts of water frequently during your workout. After exercising, drink as much water as you want. Some studies have indicated that there is no such thing as drinking too much water. Although there are many sports drinks on the market, plain water is generally the most available and least expensive replacement fluid.

Other hot weather precautions include the following: wear light-colored, loose-fitting clothing, walk during the coolest times of the day, reduce the intensity of your exercise, and reduce the duration of your exercise.

Cold Weather Walking

Dehydration can also be a problem when exercising during cold weather. When the weather is cold and dry, perspiration evaporates quickly. You should drink plenty of water and avoid diuretic liquids, such as coffee and tea.

In freezing temperatures and windy conditions, frostbite can occur within minutes on your hands, nose, ears, and toes. Be sure these areas are covered with clothing during extremely cold weather. If you are walking during cold weather and notice any tissue that is numb, or turning hard and white, take immediate action. Get indoors, where the air temperature is warmer, and soak the tissue in warm water. Do not use hot water because tissue damage may occur.

Prolonged exposure to the cold, accompanied by excessive loss of body heat, can lead to a life-threatening condition in which your core body temperature drops to a dangerous level. *Hypothermia* is the term for low body temperature. The symptoms of hypothermia include disorientation, sluggishness, slurred speech, and a stumbling gait. Be sure you dress warmly enough to maintain your core body temperature when walking during cold weather.

People with high blood pressure need to keep warm because shivering elevates blood pressure. Angina (chest pain) can also be a result of exposure to the cold. If you have angina, and the air temperature is low, wear a scarf that covers your mouth and nose. If you have any kind of cardiovascular disease, walk indoors when the outdoor temperature drops below 20° F. Mall walking has become popular, especially in colder climates.

Since cold weather is often accompanied by snow and ice, the danger of slipping and falling is increased. It is a good idea to walk where other people will be around to help in case you fall.

There is a myth that being in the cold will cause you to catch a cold. It is really viruses from others that are the primary cause of the common cold. These are most frequently found indoors, in warm, recirculated air, where we spend more time when the outside air temperature is low. Being in cold air can dry out the mucous membranes of your mouth and nose, which may make it easier for viruses to penetrate when you go indoors. Therefore, fitness walking during cold weather should not cause you to catch a cold, as long as you enter a relatively virus-free environment when you go indoors.

When exercising in cold weather, it is important to control the amount of heat lost from your body. In addition to dressing in layers of clothing, it is also important to cover your head and hands. As much as 70 percent of your body heat can be lost from these areas during cold weather if they are not covered.

As long as you are healthy and dress warmly, cold weather should not be an excuse to miss your fitness walking workout.

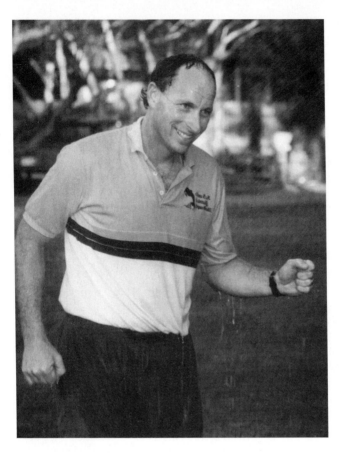

Walking in the rain can add variety to your fitness program.

Wet Weather Walking

Many beginning exercisers use wet weather as an excuse to skip their exercise session. Is this necessary? Human skin is waterproof; besides, these same people usually take a shower after exercise and get completely wet in the process. A large number of experienced fitness walkers and joggers enjoy a workout while it is raining or snowing. Remember how much fun it was to play in the rain when you were a child?

If you want to try to stay dry while walking in the rain, there are waterproof exercise suits available. Some of these water-resistant materials are expensive, but the cost is well worth it if a rain suit will help you stick with your walking program. Of course, if you walk vigorously and produce a lot of perspiration, it will not evaporate on a rainy day anyway, because the air is already completely saturated with moisture. Therefore, you will be wet from perspiration instead of rain. Walking in the rain or snow is not harmful if you take a warm bath or shower, dry off, and put on warm, dry clothing soon after you finish.

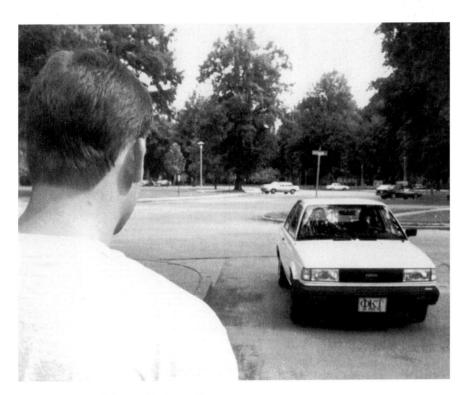
Walk on the side of the road facing traffic.

Whereas the rain does not hurt you, lightning certainly could. If there is lightning outdoors, find a way to exercise indoors.

Drugs

There is no place in a health improvement program, such as fitness walking, for the use of recreational drugs.

If you are required to take prescription drugs for your health, consult with your physician before starting an exercise program. Exercise may alter the effects of the medicine.

Cars

When a car comes near you, look directly into the driver's eyes to determine if the driver has seen you. If you suspect that the driver has not seen you, move out of the way. If a walker has a collision with an automobile, it does not matter who was right and who was wrong; the walker is the loser. Walk on the side of the road facing the oncoming traffic, and walk defensively. Make it almost impossible for a car to hit you.

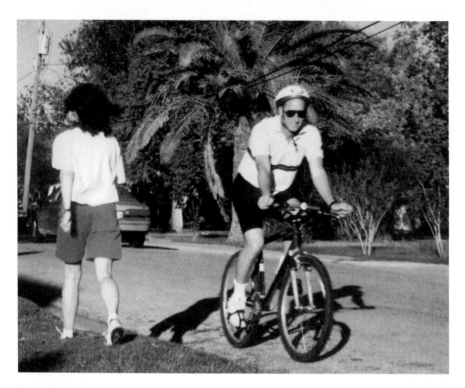

Let cyclists have the right of way.

Bicycles

Bicycle riders are supposed to obey all traffic laws; however, if you find yourself on a collision course with a bicycle, it is generally easier for you to move out of the way than it is for the person on the bicycle. Walk defensively. Don't allow a bicycle to hit you.

Dogs

No dog should have the right to decide where or when you can walk on public property. There are no guarantees that dogs will not approach you, and you have to make your own decision about what to do. Following are some ideas that have worked for others and may work for you.

If a dog comes at you, do not run away. You cannot run faster than a dog; running encourages a dog to continue the chase, and you leave yourself defenseless by turning your back toward the dog. Watch the dog but try to avoid eye contact; staring is a challenge. Do not be intimidated and do not panic. Decide what course of action is best for you. You may choose to back away slowly, but keep watching the

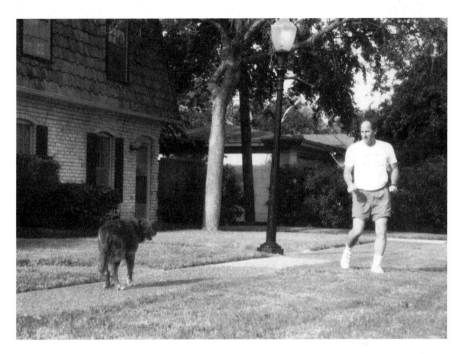

If a dog bothers you, decide what course of action is safest. It is best to avoid aggressive dogs.

dog. You may choose to walk on by slowly, or to pick up something to defend yourself, but keep watching the dog.

As a preventive measure, you might want to carry something with you when you walk, such as a protective spray or a walking stick. One idea for a walking stick is the shaft of an old golf club with the head removed. It is lightweight, sturdy, and long enough to keep dogs away.

Check the route you want to walk in a car before you walk it the first time. Walk in a group or carry some protection the first time you walk a new course. If there is an area where you want to walk and dogs are running loose, talk politely with the owners about tying them up or fencing them in during that time. Most communities have a law against dogs running loose. If the owners are not cooperative, call the dog catcher or the police. Do not give a dog the right to limit your use of public property.

Listening to Music

Listening to lively music while you fitness walk can energize your workout. However, there are safety concerns. Concentrating on the music may distract you from walking safely and the volume may prevent you from hearing traffic. Keep the volume down and watch out for traffic.

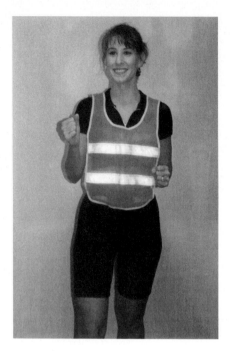

If you walk at night, wear a reflective vest or tape.

Night Walking

It is safer to walk during the daylight hours than at night; however, it is not possible for everyone to walk during the daytime, especially during winter months, when there are fewer daylight hours. If you must walk when it is dark, consider the following safety suggestions.

1. Wear light-colored clothing, a reflective vest, or reflective tape on your clothing.
2. Stay away from dark streets and alleys.
3. Walk with another person or a group.
4. Let someone know your exact route and what time you expect to be back.
5. Wear identification, including who should be called in case of an emergency and any medical conditions you have that might need to be known for proper emergency medical treatment.

Walking Surfaces

Footing is an important consideration for fitness walkers. If you are unsure of a walking surface, slow down and stay alert for dangerous spots.

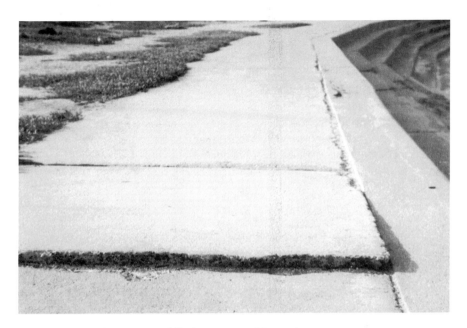

Be especially cautious on potentially dangerous walking surfaces.

When walking on pavement, watch for holes and uneven cracks that might cause you to trip. On grass, gravel, or dirt roads, watch for bumps, holes, and sudden differences in firmness. If you are walking indoors on a smooth surface, such as wood, be cautious of any wet spots; they can be extremely slippery. If you are walking on a wet or icy surface, shorten your stride, keep your knees slightly bent, and use wider than normal foot placement.

Overtraining

It is possible to get too much exercise. Exercise is a physical stressor that stimulates positive changes to take place in your body. If you exercise too much or too often, however, your body may not be able to recover. This can lead to muscle soreness, injury, illnesses, and burnout. Adequate rest and proper nutrition are essential for recovery from exercise and improvement of physical fitness.

The following are some symptoms of overtraining:

- sudden, unexpected weight loss,
- depression,
- insomnia,
- increased resting heart rate,
- decreased work capacity,
- poor performance,
- loss of enjoyment, and
- loss of motivation.

If you have been training harder and longer than usual and you have several of these symptoms, it is possible that you are overtraining. Try to get more rest between exercise sessions, watch your nutritional intake more closely, and reduce the intensity, duration, or frequency of your exercise. If the problem is overtraining, you should start to feel better within a week or two.

Each individual has a rate at which he or she can best adapt to exercise. This is not a constant rate but one that changes continually and is influenced by the other stressors in life. Although there are general guidelines for exercise, you need to listen carefully to your body to find the right amount for you.

Foot Care

The following tips will help you care for your feet.

1. Wear comfortable socks and good-quality shoes that fit properly (see chapter 3).
2. Pay close attention to hot spots on your feet. Hot spots are the first stage of a blister.
3. Keep your feet clean and dry.
4. Keep your toenails trimmed properly.
5. If you have a foot problem, go to a podiatrist.

Fitness Walking with Weights

Some fitness walkers use weights to increase the intensity of their workout. They generally add a weight vest, ankle weights, wrist weights, or hand weights. Although this may not be a problem for the advanced fitness walker, it can be dangerous for the beginner. The additional weight can interfere with the natural walking rhythm, cause unnecessary muscle soreness, and can produce an exercise load that is too great for an untrained heart.

Air Pollution

Air pollution can be a serious health problem and exercise hazard. Try to do your fitness walking in an area that has clean air. Air pollution can irritate your lungs and aggravate respiratory conditions such as asthma and bronchitis.

Noise Pollution

Noise pollution may cause additional stress, negating the psychological benefits of fitness walking. Avoid heavy construction sites, congested streets, and large airports. Plan to walk in parks, on running tracks, in quiet neighborhoods, on country roads, or in other quiet places.

Warm-Up, Cool-Down, and Flexibility

5

Warm-Up

A good warm-up before fitness walking can improve your performance and reduce your risk of injury. A proper warm-up for fitness walking requires five to ten minutes and should include slow walking and gentle stretching.

The walking portion of your warm-up should start slowly and gradually increase in speed. Your walking motion will become smoother and easier as your muscles and joints respond to the warm-up.

Stretching during the warm-up portion of your workout should be done gently and carefully. Vigorous stretching of cold muscles can result in injury and muscle soreness.

Warm-up exercises increase muscle temperature and allow your heart rate to increase gradually up to your exercise heart rate. This is a safety measure to avoid unnecessary cardiac strain.

Walk slowly for two to five minutes to warm the muscles and joints before stretching. Gradually warm up before performing vigorous physical activity.

The warm-up period is also a time to get your mind ready for exercise. It is a time to focus your attention on your workout and on the development of your body. It is a time to think about your exercise goals and what you need to do during this exercise session to help you reach those goals. Exercise is more enjoyable and more effective if you have the proper mental attitude for your training session. While you are warming up, think positive thoughts about your workout and rededicate yourself to your exercise goals.

A good warm-up should prepare you physically and mentally for the aerobic portion of your workout.

Cool-Down

The cool-down is often the most neglected portion of a workout. Many exercisers skip this part of the exercise session, thinking that the important part of the workout is finished and that the cool-down doesn't really matter. Nothing could be further from the truth.

In aviation, approximately 98 percent of all accidents occur during takeoff or landing. In general, the same is true of exercise. The time of greatest risk is usually during the transition from rest to exercise and from exercise to rest.

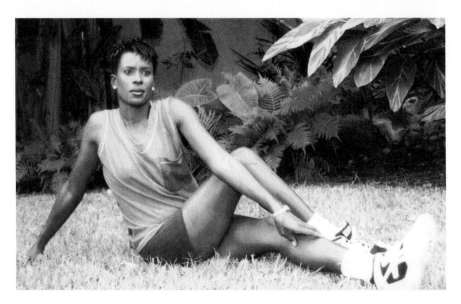
Stretching is a vital component of warming-up.

Your cool-down should generally last at least five to ten minutes and include slow walking and stretching. The more vigorous the exercise or the less fit you are, the longer it takes to cool down safely.

During the walking portion of your cool-down, there should be a gradual reduction in your speed. This will result in a gradual reduction in oxygen demand, which will allow your heart to return slowly toward its resting rate.

The rhythmic contractions of your skeletal muscles help your heart maintain adequate circulation during exercise. As your skeletal muscles contract rhythmically during walking, your veins are alternately squeezed and released. This milking action forces the blood in your veins to move toward your heart. Your blood doesn't flow back in the other direction because of blood pressure, and because of one-way valves in the veins that allow blood to flow only toward your heart. Rhythmic skeletal muscle contractions provide as much as 30 percent of the force necessary to circulate your blood during vigorous physical activity. If you stop suddenly after vigorous exercise, the important rhythmic muscle contractions also stop. Thus, blood tends to accumulate in your veins, especially in your legs. Suddenly your heart must supply 100 percent of the force necessary for circulation, a very abrupt increase in workload for your heart at a time when there is less blood returning to it. Therefore, it is recommended that you continue walking for a few minutes after the aerobic portion of your workout while gradually reducing your walking speed.

Flexibility

Flexibility is the amount of movement, or range of motion, you have at each joint. Limited range of motion of a joint can limit performance in some activities and increase the risk of injury to the body's soft tissues (muscles, tendons, and ligaments). Thus, increased flexibility is a healthy goal for most people. Stretching to improve flexibility is best done after the aerobic portion of your workout, when the soft tissues are warm and the joints are well lubricated.

General Tips for Stretching to Increase Flexibility

1. Use static stretch. To perform a static stretch, move a joint to the limit of its normal range of motion. Then, gently apply pressure to move the joint slightly beyond the point where it normally stops. Hold this position. Do not bounce. Static stretch (stretch and hold) is recommended for the following reasons: (1) it is an effective method of increasing flexibility, (2) there is less risk of injury (when compared to a "bounce type" stretch) to the soft tissues that are being stretched, (3) it helps prevent or relieve muscle soreness, (4) it is easy to learn, and (5) it can be done without a partner.

2. Stretch to the point where you feel a sensation of tightness. You should be able to feel which muscle, or group of muscles, is being stretched, but it should not be painful. Hold this position.

3. Hold each static stretch for 10 to 30 seconds. Perform each stretch one, two, or three times.

4. Do not injure the soft tissues. You should not experience extreme discomfort or pain while stretching. If you experience extreme pain, you are stretching too far.

5. Breathe slowly, rhythmically, and comfortably while stretching. Do not hold your breath. If you cannot breathe normally while stretching, you are probably stretching too far.

6. Stretch any time you feel tightness. Stretching does not have to be restricted to your workout.

7. Warm-up stretches with cold muscles and joints should be light and easy.

8. Be sure your muscles are completely warmed up before performing stretching exercises to increase flexibility. Walk for a few minutes after you have completed the aerobic portion of your workout to allow your heart rate to return toward a resting level. Then stretch your muscles. They will stay warm for a long time after exercise.

9. Make stretching a relaxing daily habit. Some people like to stretch when they get up in the morning. It makes them feel better. Some people like to stretch before going to bed. It helps them relax and sleep well. Some people stretch before and after their daily exercise. It improves their performance and reduces their risk of injury.

Four Standing Stretches for Fitness Walking

Many fitness walkers do not stretch before and after walking. They say it takes too long, they don't feel like they have an appropriate place to stretch, and they don't want to sit down or lay down or get dirty. One solution is to combine stretching exercises and do them from a standing position.

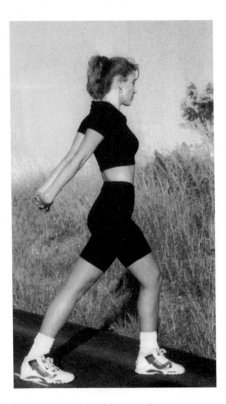

The lunge and shoulder stretch.

Stretch Number One—Lunge and Shoulder Stretch

- Head and trunk erect
- One leg back
- Back foot pointing straight ahead, heel on ground
- Top of hips tilted back, low back flat
- Back knee straight 15 seconds, bent 15 seconds
- Front knee bent
- Hands behind back, fingers interlaced
- Elbows as straight as possible
- Arms raised as high as possible
- Hold 10 to 30 seconds
- Change legs and hold 10 to 30 seconds
- Feel the stretch in the ankle of your back foot, back of your lower leg, front of your hip joint, front of your shoulder joint, and chest

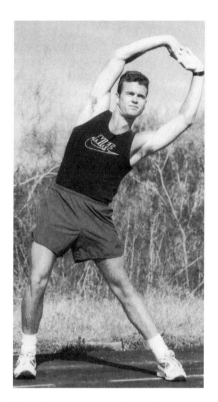

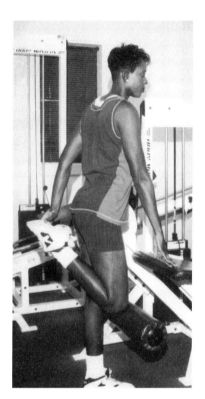

The adductor, trunk, and shoulder stretch.

The standing quadricep stretch.

Stretch Number Two—Adductor, Trunk, and Shoulder Stretch

- Feet wide apart (2 to 3 times shoulder width)
- Hands together overhead, palms facing up
- Bend your right knee
- Lean toward your left
- Feel stretch in your right shoulder, right side of your trunk, and your left adductor group (inside of your left thigh)
- Hold 10 to 30 seconds
- Change sides, bend your left knee and lean toward your right side
- Hold 10 to 30 seconds

Stretch Number Three—Standing Quadricep Stretch

- Bend your right knee
- Hold the toes of your right foot with your left hand
- Feel the stretch on the front of your lower leg, front of your thigh, and front of your hip
- Hold 10 to 30 seconds
- Change sides, hold the toes of your left foot with your right hand
- Hold 10 to 30 seconds

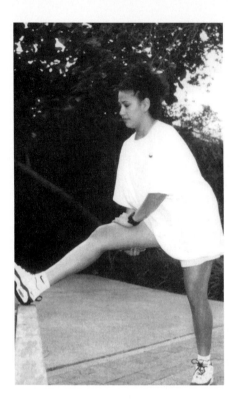

The hamstring and low back stretch.

Stretch Number Four—Standing Hamstring and Low Back Stretch

- Place the heel of your right foot on a low step or bench (appropriate for your flexibility)
- Place both hands on your right thigh above your knee
- Gently bend forward at your hip and waist with your right knee slightly bent
- Feel the gentle stretch in the back of your thigh and your lower back
- Maintain a slight bend in your support leg
- Hold 10 to 30 seconds
- Change legs and hold 10 to 30 seconds

**Refer to Activity 5a
in the back of this book.**

Fitness Walking Test(s)

6

What is your present cardiovascular fitness level? This chapter will describe two walking tests you can use to measure your cardiovascular fitness level. Both tests are one mile long.

Knowing your current fitness level can help you find a realistic place to start your fitness walking program. By starting at the appropriate exercise level, you will find that your walking program will be safer, more productive, and more enjoyable.

If you have been sedentary, be very cautious about taking any fitness test. Do not push yourself too hard during the test. It is much safer to complete the test comfortably and be classified in a lower fitness category than to push yourself too hard and risk injury. Some experts recommend beginning with a low-intensity starter program for at least two or three weeks before taking any fitness test.

Many people start exercise programs every year with unrealistic expectations. They start out highly motivated and full of enthusiasm, but with little knowledge of their present fitness level or of the amount of exercise they need. Consequently, they frequently start out doing too much. This often leads to muscle soreness, extreme fatigue, frustration, injury, or burnout. As a result, most of these people lose their motivation and quit exercising.

It is unrealistic to think you can make up for years of bad habits in a few days. The benefits of regular exercise come from a lifetime habit of moderate exercise. It is better to start at a comfortable level of fitness walking and enjoy it for the rest of your life than to exercise at a high level for a few days and quit.

To prevent this from occurring, test yourself. This will enable you to start a fitness walking program that will best fit your needs and present physical condition. You will be able to enjoy your walking program while you progress gradually and safely.

Before taking the fitness walking tests, make sure it is medically safe for you to participate. Review the discussion of medical clearance in chapter 4 and complete Activity 4a before taking either the Rockport Fitness Walking Test or the One-Mile Walk Test.

Why the Rockport Fitness Walking Test?

Researchers at the University of Massachusetts Medical School found that cardiovascular fitness can be estimated fairly accurately using four factors: age, gender, time to walk one mile, and heart rate at the completion of a one-mile walk. The researchers developed charts for estimating cardiovascular fitness level using these

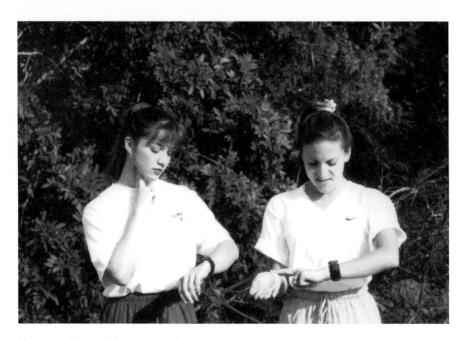

Use either the carotid artery or radial artery to count your pulse.

four factors and fitness norms from the American Heart Association. This field test of cardiovascular fitness is called the Rockport Fitness Walking Test.

How to Take the Rockport Fitness Walking Test

To take the Rockport Fitness Walking Test, you need to be able to count your heart rate. Gently place the fingertips of your index finger and middle finger on the radial artery. You will find this artery on the palm side of your forearm, just above your wrist. You can also count your pulse by placing the same two fingertips on the carotid artery. You will find this artery by placing your fingertips along the side of your trachea near the top.

To take the walking test, you need a watch that can measure time in minutes and seconds. Find a flat, measured mile to walk. A quarter-mile track is an excellent place. If there is not a track available, measure a one-mile course where you can walk continuously. Avoid traffic and stoplights. It is a good idea to measure a half mile so you can walk out and back. That way, you will know when you are halfway through the test and you will end up back where you started.

Walk the mile as fast as you can while maintaining a constant pace. Running is not allowed. However, think safety first. Do not endanger your health. Slow down if the pace is too severe.

Two measurements are necessary to determine your current fitness level. One is the number of minutes and seconds it takes you to walk one mile. The other is your heart rate immediately after finishing the mile. Obviously, speeding up or slowing down near the end of the test will affect your heart rate, walking time, and test results. Maintain a steady pace.

When you cross the finish line, record your time in minutes and seconds. Within five seconds after you finish, locate your pulse and count the number of pulse beats in 15 seconds. Multiply this number by four to get your exercise heart rate in beats per minute. The reason for locating your pulse immediately and taking a 15-second pulse count is to find your exercise heart rate. A great deal of recovery can occur within the first minute after you stop exercising; therefore, if you wait too long to locate your pulse, or take a longer count, your test results will not be valid.

How to Find Your Fitness Category

Once your results are recorded you can determine your current fitness level by looking at the appropriate fitness level chart for your age and gender.

On the horizontal line at the top of the chart, locate your time to complete the one-mile walk. Place a mark on the line at that point.

On the vertical line on the left side of the chart locate your exercise heart rate in beats per minute. Place a mark on the line at that point.

Draw a line straight down from your time and another line straight across from your heart rate. The point at which the two lines intersect indicates your cardiovascular fitness level.

The relative fitness charts for 20–29-year-olds can be used for individuals under the age of 20. Recent research has indicated that this test tends to overpredict the cardiovascular fitness category of individuals under the age of 30 as compared to other measures of cardiovascular fitness. At this time research work is continuing in the following areas: (1) new prediction equations for people under the age 30, (2) a fitness walking test that would use age, gender, and time but not heart rate, and (3) a two-kilometer walking test. However, for now, if the results of the Rockport Fitness Walking Test place you in a beginning walking program that is too difficult—change to an easier program.

Interpreting the Results

What do your results mean? To understand your performance on the test, let's use as an example a 22-year-old woman who scored in the level 4 fitness category. Her results indicate that she is above average in cardiovascular fitness when compared to other women of her age group (20–29).

Retesting

How often should you retest yourself on the Rockport Fitness Walking Test? Ideally, it is best to wait until you finish a 20-week fitness walking program as outlined in

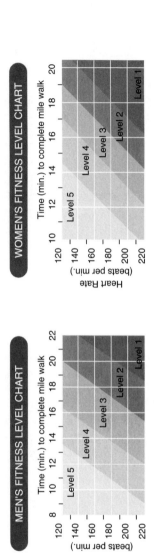

AGE 20-29

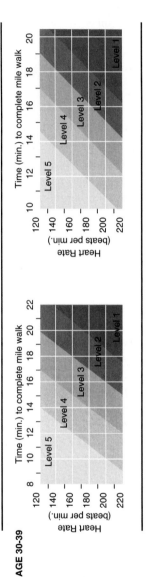

AGE 30-39

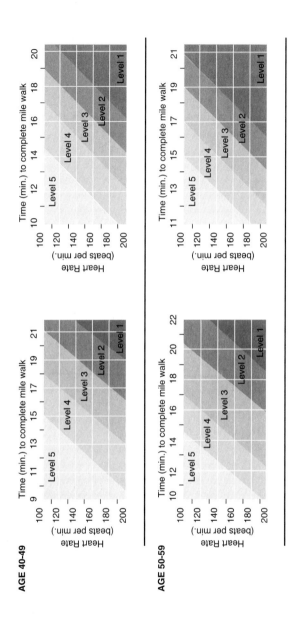

AGE 40-49

Time (min.) to complete mile walk

Heart Rate (beats per min.)

Level 5 Level 4 Level 3 Level 2 Level 1

AGE 50-59

Time (min.) to complete mile walk

Heart Rate (beats per min.)

Level 5 Level 4 Level 3 Level 2 Level 1

MEN'S FITNESS LEVEL CHART

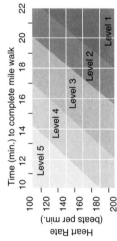

WOMEN'S FITNESS LEVEL CHART

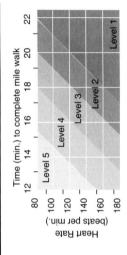

chapter 7. The most important benefits come from a consistent and lifelong fitness walking program. By retesting yourself too frequently, you tend to focus your attention on short-term changes. Although short-term changes are interesting, the long-term benefits are more important.

When you retest after completing a 20-week fitness walking program, you may find that you have moved up to another fitness level. If that is the case, base your next fitness walking program on your new fitness level.

When you reach the point where you are satisfied with your cardiovascular fitness level, change to a maintenance walking program. Taking the walking test two or three times a year should be sufficient once you are on a maintenance program; however, some regular walkers prefer to take the test once a month. This helps them monitor their fitness level on a regular basis and provides motivation for them to keep up with their exercise program.

Refer to Activities 6a and 6b
in the back of this book.

The One-Mile Walk Test

Another walking test is the One-Mile Walk Test (table 6.1). Dr. James Rippe of the University of Massachusetts designed a One-Mile Walk Test to evaluate aerobic fitness. If you have been physically inactive, it's a good idea to consult with your physician before taking this walk test.

Directions: Either time yourself or get a partner to time you walking a mile as fast as you can. Compare your time with the following chart. This will estimate your current level of fitness. Then, check in the section entitled The One-Mile Walk Program in chapter 7 to discover what walking program is best for you to follow based on your fitness category.

Table 6.1   The One-Mile Walk Test

Fitness Category	Female (min.:sec.)	Male (min.:sec.)
Excellent	Less than 11:40	Less than 10:12
Good/High	11:41–13:08	10:13–11:42
Average	13:09–14:36	11:43–13:13
Low/Average	14:37–16:04	13:14–14:44
Fair	16:05–17:31	14:45–16:23
Poor	More than 17:31	More than 16:23

Fitness Walking Programs

7

Exercise is like medicine. Both can be good for you if you get the right type and the right amount. Fitness walking is the right type of exercise for most people. This chapter will help you select the right amount. In this chapter you will find four different ways to get started on a walking program: the Rockport programs, the One-Mile Walk program, the American Heart Association program, and information to design your own program.

Rockport Walking Programs

If you have completed the Rockport Fitness Walking Test you are ready to select your fitness walking program. The Rockport Walking Programs (page 56–58) correspond to your current cardiovascular fitness level as measured by the Rockport Fitness Walking Test.

The Rockport Walking Programs were developed by the cardiologists and exercise scientists at the University of Massachusetts Medical School. They are designed to improve or maintain your current level of fitness. For best results, follow the programs closely.

At the end of each 20-week period, retake the Rockport Fitness Walking Test to determine your new fitness level and exercise program.

On each program, you will see columns labeled "Pace" and "Heart Rate." The pace listed is only an approximation. Walking speed should be the pace that keeps your heart rate at the appropriate percentage listed.

A Walking Program Based on the One-Mile Walk Test

Always begin and end each walk with 2 to 5 minutes of low-intensity walking and stretching exercises for the muscles of your arms, chest, back, hips, and legs. Design your walking routine according to your present fitness level, as determined by the One-Mile Walk Test in chapter 6. Always consult with your physician before beginning any exercise program.

Level 1

WEEK	1–2	3–4	5	6	7–8	9	10	11	12–13	14	15–16	17–18	19–20
WARM-UP/COOL DOWN (stretches before and after walk in min.)	5–7	5–7	5–7	5–7	5–7	5–7	5–7	5–7	5–7	5–7	5–7	5–7	5–7
MILEAGE	1.0	1.25	1.5	1.5	1.75	2.0	2.0	2.0	2.25	2.5	2.5	2.75	3.0
PACE (MPH)	3.0	3.0	3.0	3.5	3.5	3.5	3.75	3.75	3.75	3.75	4.0	4.0	4.0
HEART RATE (% OF MAX)	60	60	60	60–70	60–70	60–70	60–70	70	70	70	70	70–80	70–80
FREQUENCY (TIMES PER WEEK)	5	5	5	5	5	5	5	5	5	5	5	5	5

Level 2

WEEK	1–2	3–4	5–6	7	8–9	10–12	13	14	15–16	17–18	19–20
WARM-UP/COOL DOWN (stretches before and after walk in min.)	5–7	5–7	5–7	5–7	5–7	5–7	5–7	5–7	5–7	5–7	5–7
MILEAGE	1.5	1.75	2.0	2.0	2.25	2.5	2.75	2.75	3.0	3.25	3.5
PACE (MPH)	3.0	3.0	3.0	3.5	3.5	3.5	3.5	4.0	4.0	4.0	4.0
HEART RATE (% OF MAX)	60–70	60–70	60–70	70	70	70	70–80	70–80	70–80	70–80	70–80
FREQUENCY (TIMES PER WEEK)	5	5	5	5	5	5	5	5	5	5	5

Level 3

WEEK	1	2	3–4	5	6–8	9–10	11–12	13–14	15	16–17	18–20	maintenance
WARM-UP/COOL DOWN (stretches before and after walk in min.)	5–7	5–7	5–7	5–7	5–7	5–7	5–7	5–7	5–7	5–7	5–7	5–7
MILEAGE	2.0	2.25	2.5	2.75	2.75	3.0	3.0	3.25	3.5	3.5	4.0	4.0
PACE (MPH)	3.0	3.0	3.0	3.0	3.5	3.5	4.0	4.0	4.0	4.5	4.5	4.5
HEART RATE (% OF MAX)	70	70	70	70	70	70	70–80	70–80	70–80	70–80	70–80	70–80
FREQUENCY (TIMES PER WEEK)	5	5	5	5	5	5	5	5	5	5	5	3–5

Level 4

WEEK	1	2	3–4	5	6	7	8	9–10	11–14	15–20	maintenance
WARM-UP/COOL DOWN (stretches before and after walk in min.)	5–7	5–7	5–7	5–7	5–7	5–7	5–7	5–7	5–7	5–7	5–7
MILEAGE	2.5	2.75	3.0	3.25	3.5	3.5	3.75	4.0	4.0	4.0	4.0
PACE (MPH)	3.5	3.5	3.5	3.5	3.5	4.0	4.0	4.0	4.5	4.5	4.5
HEART RATE (% OF MAX)	70	70	70	70	70–80	70–80	70–80	70–80	70–80	70–80	70–80
FREQUENCY (TIMES PER WEEK)	5	5	5	5	5	5	5	5	5	5	5

Level 5

WEEK	1	2	3	4	5	6	7–20	maintenance
WARM-UP/COOL DOWN (stretches before and after walk in min.)	5–7	5–7	5–7	5–7	5–7	5–7	5–7	5–7
MILEAGE	3.0	3.25	3.5	3.5	3.75	4.0	4.0	4.0
PACE (MPH)	4.0	4.0	4.0	4.5	4.5	4.5	4.5	4.5
HEART RATE (% OF MAX)	70	70	70	70–80	70–80	70–80	70–80	70–80
FREQUENCY (TIMES PER WEEK)	5	5	5	5	5	5	5	3–5

Guidelines for Planning Your Own Personal Fitness Walking Programs

The Rockport Fitness Walking Programs are excellent; however, some walkers may want to plan their own fitness walking program. The following guidelines will help you plan your own program.

The Right Amount of Exercise

The right amount of exercise is determined by the characteristics of frequency, intensity, time, and type (FITT).

Frequency

How often should you walk? Fitness walking must be performed regularly to be effective. The recommended frequency for fitness walking is three to seven days per week.

Intensity

How fast do you need to walk? Intensity refers to how hard you need to exercise to benefit from each training session. Exercise heart rate provides an indication of how hard you are exercising. A guideline for fitness walking is to reach an exercise heart rate that is between 60 and 90 percent of your maximum heart rate. To estimate your maximum heart rate, subtract your age from 220.

Beginning fitness walkers should start out at a low intensity, 60 to 70 percent of their maximum heart rate. Only advanced fitness walkers should attempt to exercise at a higher intensity—80 to 90 percent of their maximum heart rate.

Some people believe the old athletic myth of "no pain, no gain." It is not true. They actually believe that you must exercise until you are in pain for exercise to be beneficial. Of course, this is one of the reasons they do not exercise regularly. Normal people avoid painful experiences.

> **Refer to Activity 7a
> in the back of this book.**

Time

How long do you need to walk? You should walk for 20 to 60 minutes at your prescribed exercise heart rate. If you are just starting a fitness walking program, keep the intensity low and the duration short. Gradually increase the duration first, then the intensity.

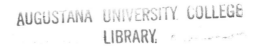

Type

Why is fitness walking the right type of exercise? Fitness walking is considered the right type of exercise because it is aerobic. Aerobic exercises develop cardiovascular fitness, reduce cardiovascular disease, and help lower body fat. These benefits are a result of using large muscle groups rhythmically and continuously. This causes the body to use larger amounts of oxygen and calories for an extended period of time.

Guidelines for Fitness Walking to Develop Cardiovascular Fitness

F.I.T.T.

Frequency	Three to seven days per week
Intensity	60 to 90 percent of maximum heart rate
Time	20 to 60 minutes
Type	Aerobic exercise (fitness walking)

Recovery

How much exercise is too much? As a general guideline, if you experience extreme muscle soreness the next day and cannot repeat your fitness walking workout, you have done too much and need to reduce the amount of exercise the next time.

Exercise is only the stimulus for positive biological changes to occur in your body. These changes actually occur during the recovery time between exercise sessions. Make sure the exercise stimulus is not too severe and that you get adequate rest and nutrition between walking workouts.

A problem for some middle-aged people is that they want to get back into the physical condition they were in when they were young. This is not a realistic expectation. Many people who have been inactive for a long time want to get in shape quickly; however, biological adaptation is a relatively slow process. You cannot expect to reverse the effects of years of sedentary living in a few days or weeks. These people often fall into the trap of thinking that, if a little exercise is good, then more must be better. This is only true to a point. Beyond that point, additional exercise can be harmful. Follow the exercise guidelines. Progress slowly and safely. If you try to progress too quickly, you are likely to become injured. When you are injured, you are likely to lose your motivation to exercise. If you lose your motivation and quit, you will not achieve the benefits that come from regular exercise.

If you are exercising for your health, you do not need to improve forever. When you reach the fitness level you want, change to a walking program that will keep you at that level.

These guidelines will help you select and maintain a safe and enjoyable walking program that you can stay with and benefit from for the rest of your life.

Because there is less to keep track of, some people prefer creating their own program rather than using the Rockport program. If you follow these guidelines, all you

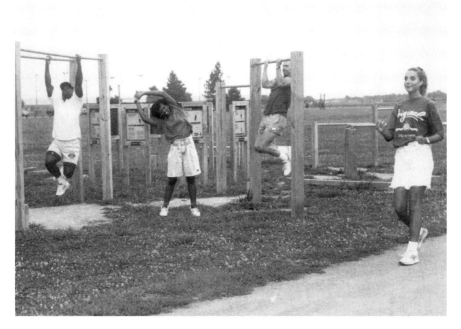

Total fitness includes cardiovascular endurance, muscular endurance, strength, flexibility, and body composition.

need to keep track of is your total minutes walked at your exercise heart rate. This method also gives you greater freedom to walk new courses, since you do not need to know the exact distance.

American Heart Association Walking Program

The American Heart Association offers a program that is safe for most beginners. Each workout should consist of a warm-up, a walk within the target heart rate zone, and a cool-down. You are encouraged to keep your exercise heart rate between 60 and 75 percent of your maximum heart rate and walk at least three times each week.

Total Health-Related Physical Fitness

Total health-related physical fitness includes cardiovascular endurance, muscular endurance, strength, flexibility, and body composition.

Cardiovascular Endurance

Cardiovascular endurance refers to your ability to continue vigorous total body activity for a relatively long period of time. As mentioned previously, to develop

Week	Target Zone Exercising	Total Time in Minutes (warm-up + target zone exercising + cool-down)
1	Walk briskly 5 min.	15 min.
2	Walk briskly 7 min.	17 min.
3	Walk briskly 9 min.	19 min.
4	Walk briskly 11 min.	21 min.
5	Walk briskly 13 min.	23 min.
6	Walk briskly 15 min.	25 min.
7	Walk briskly 18 min.	28 min.
8	Walk briskly 20 min.	30 min.
9	Walk briskly 23 min.	33 min.
10	Walk briskly 26 min.	36 min.
11	Walk briskly 28 min.	38 min.
12	Walk briskly 30 min.	40 min.
13 on:	Check your pulse periodically to see if you are exercising within your target zone. As you get more in shape, try exercising within the upper range of your target heart zone. Remember that your goal is to continue getting the benefits you seek while enjoying your activity.	

Reproduced with permission. WALKING FOR A HEALTHY HEART, American Heart Association.

cardiovascular endurance, you should perform exercises that use large muscle groups rhythmically and continuously. Maintain an exercise heart rate that is 60 to 90 percent of your maximum heart rate for 20 to 60 minutes, and repeat this workout three to seven times each week.

Muscle Endurance

Muscle endurance refers to the ability of individual muscles or muscle groups to exert force for many repetitions or to hold a position for an extended period of time. To develop muscle endurance, perform exercises that require movement through a full range of motion against resistance. Use a resistance that is 50 to 70 percent of your maximum voluntary contraction (the heaviest you can lift at one time) and execute 20 to 30 repetitions. Perform one to three sets of each exercise and repeat your muscle endurance exercises three to five days per week.

Strength

Strength refers to the amount of force a muscle can exert. To develop strength, perform exercises that involve movement through a full range of motion against resistance. Use a resistance that is 70 to 100 percent of your maximum voluntary contraction (the most weight you can lift at one time) and execute 1 to 10 repetitions. Perform each exercise for one to three sets and repeat your strength training program three days per week.

Flexibility

To develop flexibility, use static stretch exercises. Stretch to the point where you feel a sensation of tightness, and hold each stretch for 15 to 30 seconds. Perform each stretch one to three times, and repeat your stretching program three to seven days per week.

Body Composition

Body composition refers to the amount of muscle, fat, bone, and other tissues that makes up the body. The best exercises to develop healthy levels of body fat are those that use large muscle groups rhythmically and continuously. Exercise at a heart rate that is 60 to 80 percent of your estimated heart rate range for 30 to 60 minutes and repeat this workout five to seven days per week.

A Total Health-Related Physical Fitness Program

Fitness walking programs, including the stretching exercises during the warm-up and cool-down, develop cardiovascular endurance, muscular endurance, flexibility, and a healthy body fat level. Adding a few strength exercises after the walking portion, and before the stretching portion of your cool-down results in a good total health-related physical fitness program.

A total health-related physical fitness walking program is as follows:

- Warm-up walking
- Gentle stretch
- Fitness walking at exercise heart rate
- Cool-down walking
- Strength and muscle endurance exercises
- Cool-down stretching (flexibility stretching)

Fitness Walking Techniques

8

This chapter explains some specific walking techniques that will increase your speed, stride length, and efficiency. As you acquire new skills, you should also improve your balance, coordination, body control, posture, and agility.

Once you have learned the proper form of fitness walking, your pace will become faster. Your heart and lungs will work harder to supply the oxygen needed by the working muscles. This will improve your cardiovascular conditioning.

Even after you have learned these walking techniques and have become a skilled fitness walker, you may want to return to this chapter to review the techniques. Even the most experienced fitness walkers continue to review and improve their walking form.

Learn one walking technique at a time, focusing on one each workout. After practicing each technique until it becomes natural, combine them to become a highly skilled fitness walker.

Technique 1: Posture and Alignment

For the smoothest walking motion, maintain correct posture and body alignment. Apply the guidelines in Activity 8a while you walk.

> **Refer to Activity 8a
> in the back of this book.**

Technique 2: Heel Contact

From a position of correct posture, swing one leg forward. Land on your heel, with the bottom of your foot at about a 40-degree angle to the ground. Do not land flat-footed or on the ball of your foot.

> **Refer to Activity 8b
> in the back of this book.**

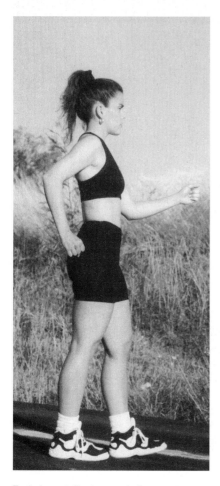

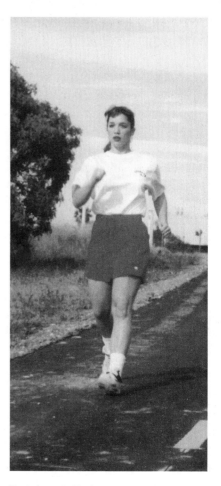

Technique 1: Posture and alignment.   Technique 2: Heel contact.

Technique 3: Heel-to-Toe Roll

Once your heel makes contact with the ground, begin to roll your foot forward, keeping your weight slightly toward the outer edge of your foot until reaching your toes. The outer edge of your foot acts as a natural rocker bottom for continuous forward motion. As you roll your foot forward with your weight toward the outer edge, keep your knees pointing straight ahead.

**Refer to Activity 8c
in the back of this book.**

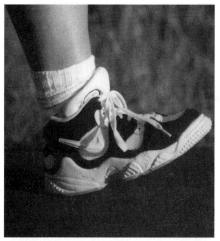 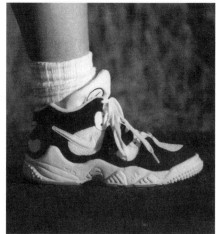

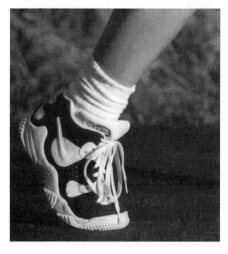

Technique 3: Heel-to-toe roll.

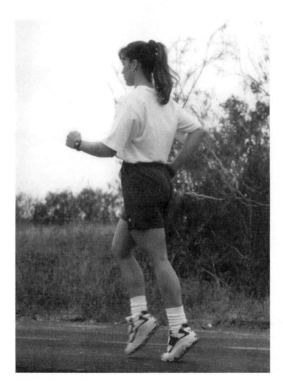

Technique 4: Push-off.

Technique 4: Push-Off

Following the heel-to-toe roll, continue your forward motion with a push-off from your toes. Resist the temptation to pick up your foot early, as you might do in casual walking. Keep your foot in contact with the ground for as long as possible. You can lengthen your stride on each step by pushing off with your toes.

To reduce excessive side-to-side swaying and undue stress on your joints, keep your support foot pointing straight ahead. If your body rises and falls with each step, you may be pushing off from the front part of your foot instead of your toes. If this happens, reduce your speed and focus on the push-off.

To receive the greatest benefits from fitness walking, it is necessary to walk at a brisk pace.

Stretching exercises are recommended to improve your ankle, foot, and toe flexibility for a greater range of motion on the push-off.

> **Refer to Activity 8d
> in the back of this book.**

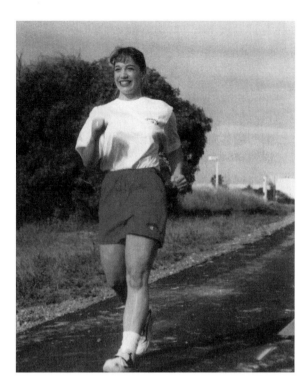

Technique 5: Arm swing.

Technique 5: Arm Swing

The arms play an important role in fitness walking. Your arms and legs are like team-mates—the faster you swing your arms, the faster your legs will move.

During fitness walking, your arms should be bent at about a 90-degree angle at the elbow joint. Your hands should be in a relaxed fist position, with your palms facing inward. In this position, your arms should swing forward and backward from the shoulder joint. Each arm should swing in a natural path and remain fairly close to your body to avoid side-to-side swaying of your upper body and hips. On the for-ward swing, your hand should rise to the level of the xiphoid process at the bottom of the sternum (where the ribs join at the bottom of the chest). On the backswing your hand should stop at the waist/hip area.

**Refer to Activity 8e
in the back of this book.**

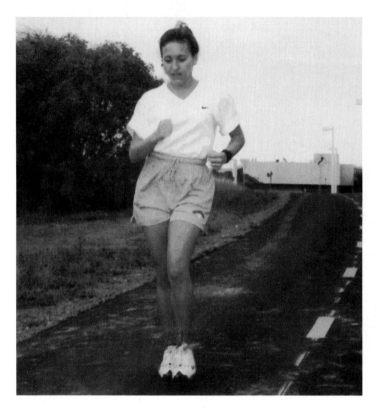

Technique 6: Hip movement.

Technique 6: Hip Movement

Keep your back foot in contact with the ground until you have full extension of your leg and you push off from your toes. When swinging your leg to the front, reach forward with your front foot as far as comfort will allow. This technique alone can add as much as eight inches to your stride length.

Using the hips more reduces the amount of up-and-down movement with each step, converting wasted vertical energy into useful horizontal energy. Also, the abdominal and hip muscles are exercised more vigorously with increased hip movement.

**Refer to Activity 8f
in the back of this book.**

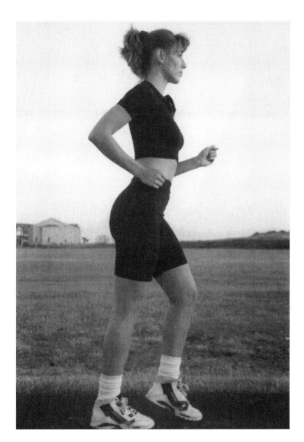

Technique 7: Leg vault.

Technique 7: Leg Vault

Incorporating the leg vault technique into your walking movement will add even more forward drive to your push-off. For this technique, it is helpful to think of your support leg as a vaulting pole. Heel contact is the pole plant of fitness walking. Swing one leg forward. At the point of contact, your leg should be straight, but not rigidly locked into extension at the knee. The idea is to reach out with the front leg and make contact with the ground, using the longest practical stride.

Vault your body forward, using your support leg as a vaulting pole. Finish the vaulting action with your leg extended and a final push-off from your toes before bending at the knee and swinging your leg forward.

> **Refer to Activity 8g
> in the back of this book.**

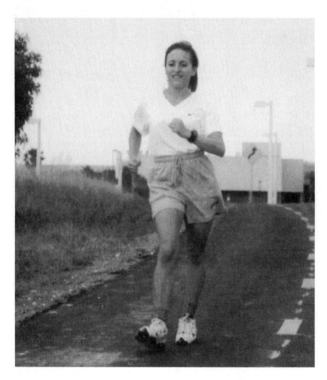

Technique 8: Racewalk.

Technique 8: The Racewalk

Racewalking is an advanced skill that requires accelerated arm and leg speed. Walk tall, relax, and feel your body's action. You want to stay loose through the pelvis and hips and thrust each hip forward to achieve optimum stride length. To racewalk, you must swing your arms and legs quickly. This is an extremely tiring technique. You will need to build up your time and distance gradually using this all-out speed.

Two rules must be followed to prevent disqualification in competition. Racewalkers must keep one foot in contact with the ground at all times, and the support leg must be straight (not bent at the knee) in the vertical position.

Racewalking is not for beginners; it is for intermediate and advanced fitness walkers who want a higher-intensity workout. Racewalking could result in very sore muscles or injury for unconditioned beginners.

**Refer to Activity 8h
in the back of this book.**

Fitness Walking Techniques

1. Posture and alignment
2. Heel contact
3. Heel-to-toe roll
4. Push-off
5. Arm swing
6. Hip movement
7. Leg vault
8. The racewalk

Tips for Higher-Intensity Workouts

Once you have mastered the basic fitness walking techniques and have developed your cardiovascular fitness to a high level, you may find it difficult to reach your training heart rate. The following section will highlight some other ideas besides racewalking to help you increase your workout intensity. High-intensity workouts should not be used by beginners.

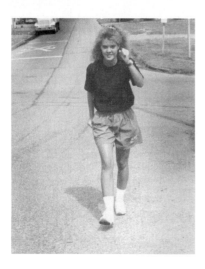

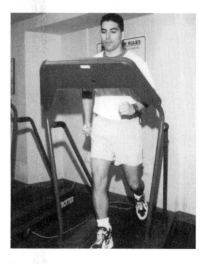

Hill walking.

Treadmill walking.

Hill Walking

Hill walking will increase your exercise intensity and add variety to your walking routine. It will also improve your cardiovascular fitness level. Depending on the steepness of the hill, your heart rate will be 10 to 50 beats per minute higher when walking uphill. This increase in exercise heart rate makes hill walking an excellent cardiovascular conditioner and a great calorie burner.

Treadmill Walking

During extreme weather conditions and at all hours of the day and night, treadmills are an excellent substitute for a walk outdoors. Treadmills offer the walker a safe walking surface and the ability to control speed and elevation. Many walkers use treadmills to complement their normal walking programs, whereas others depend on them exclusively.

Stair Walking

Stair walking is hill walking for those who do not have hills. It is a superb exercise for the cardiovascular system. In addition to the aerobic benefits, stair walking develops muscular strength in your legs and hips, since your body weight must be lifted with each step. To increase your exercise intensity and add variety to your fitness walking program, try stair walking.

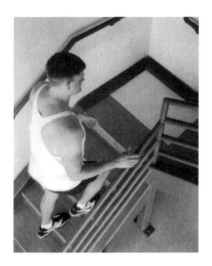

Stair walking.

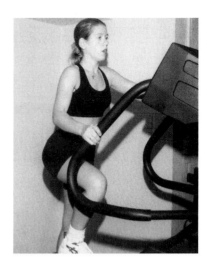

Stair walking.

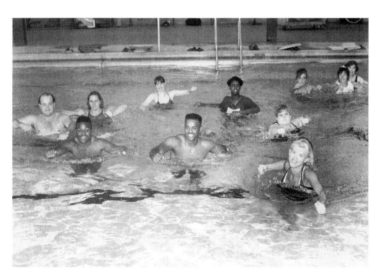

Water walking.

Water Walking

Especially during the hot weather months, walking in deep water offers the triple bonus of exercise, less shock impact, and a refreshing environment. When music is added, the water walker feels even more ready to swing those legs and pump those arms. Striding through the water provides a cardiovascular workout, and can use more calories than land walking. At three miles an hour in thigh-deep water, you will use approximately 460 calories versus 240 for land walking. Next time you're at a pool, give water walking a try.

Strategies for Healthy Nutrition

9

"Balance, variety, and moderation—the formula for healthy eating!"

Introduction

Each day we have many choices to make about food: when to eat, what to eat, and how much to eat. We also all have to eat and drink to stay alive. This is one lifestyle behavior that is mandatory. The key is to eat and drink for energy and health, not just because food tastes good or is convenient. Experts are in agreement that our eating patterns play a major role in our level of well-being.

Nutrition experts agree that healthy nutrition is built upon balance, variety, and moderation. This means enjoying many different foods in moderate portions without giving up your favorite selections. A healthy diet can prevent the consumption of too many calories, too much of any one nutrient, or too much of any single food.

The college years often bring about changes in food patterns. Factors such as class attendance, long study hours, work, finances, and extracurricular activities can interfere with healthy eating patterns. As a result of busy schedules, college students become more dependent on fast foods, delivery services, and vending machines to satisfy appetite and supply energy.

What Is Nutrition?

Nutrition comes from the Latin word that means *to nourish,* or providing all that is necessary to sustain life. Human nutrition, therefore, is defined as the science of food, the study of its uses within the body, and its relationship to health. Proper nutrition sustains life by promoting good health.

The study of nutrition involves knowing about approximately 46 essential nutrients, which fall into six major categories: **carbohydrates, fats, proteins, vitamins, minerals,** and **water.** Nutrition is concerned with how the body utilizes these nutrients and their effects upon your health. Positive nutritional behavior includes choosing the daily recommended servings from the Food Guide Pyramid and following the dietary guidelines recommended for Americans by the U.S. Department of Agriculture.

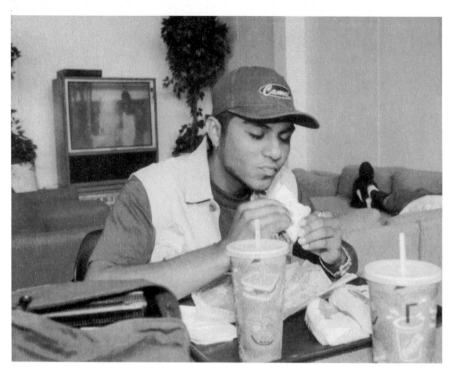

Over time your eating selections become cumulative.

Nutrition and Wellness

Proper nutrition has long been considered an important factor contributing to a healthy lifestyle. Positive nutritional practices can enhance growth, development, and optimal health. In addition, eating well can improve vitality, enhance quality of life, and lead to greater life expectancy. On the other hand, unhealthy nutritional behaviors such as high-fat diets can be a contributing factor to such problems as heart disease, cancer, stroke, diabetes, obesity, gallstones, and arthritis.

Although the act of eating is a voluntary activity, it becomes habitual because it is given little thought. More than a thousand times a year, you choose to eat a meal. In your lifetime, you will consume more than seventy thousand meals. Imagine how many thousands of pounds of food that is! In one day, your eating selections may affect your health only slightly, but in the long term they become cumulative.

Most people need to distinguish between **hunger** and **appetite.** Hunger is the physiological need for food, while appetite is the desire to eat. The physiological need by your body for food is often satisfied much sooner than is your appetite. In order to promote good health, we need to learn to control appetite. There is, indeed, some truth in the saying, "Always leave the table a little hungry."

Food affects all dimensions of wellness. Most people view food as only affecting the physical dimension of wellness, when actually it influences all dimensions (see figure 9.1). To a large degree, our social dimension is centered around food—not

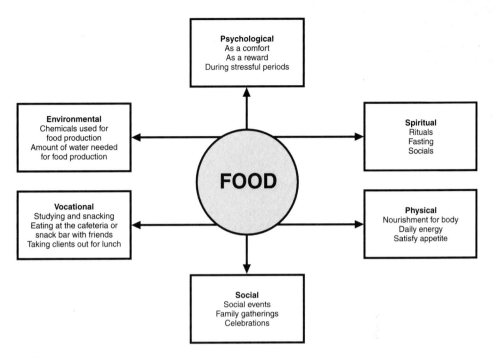

Figure 9.1
Food affects all wellness components.

around nutrition. The good host offers guests something to eat and drink. What, for instance, would a party or casual get-together be like without food or drink? Food can be used also to comfort us emotionally when we are sad or upset, or it can be used as a reward during happy times. These are a few examples of the importance of food in society.

Calories (Kilocalories)

The term **Calorie** is used to indicate the energy-producing value of food when oxidized in the body. When discussing nutrition, we use *Calorie* (with a capital C), which is actually a **kilocalorie (kcal),** and is defined as the amount of heat (or energy) required to raise the temperature of 1 *kilogram* (or 1000 grams) of water by 1 degree Celsius. If an apple, therefore, contains a hundred Calories, it provides a hundred units of energy. See table 9.1 for the caloric values of nutrients and how they apply to each nutrient.

The Six Classes of Nutrients

The six classes of nutrients are carbohydrates, fats, proteins, vitamins, minerals, and water (see figure 9.2). Basically, nutrients perform three functions. First, nutrients

Table 9.1 The Caloric Value of Nutrients

Nutrient	Calories
1 gram of protein	4
1 gram of carbohydrates (sugar or starch)	4
1 gram of alcohol	7
1 gram of fat	9
Vitamins, minerals, water, fiber	0

How to Apply the Caloric Value to Each Nutrient

A serving of microwave popping corn (3 cups popped) contains 17 grams of carbohydrate, 3 grams of protein, 8 grams of fat, and 152 calories.

Carbohydrate:

17 grams × 4 calories per gram = calories from carbohydrate (68 ÷152 = 45%)

Protein:

3 grams × 4 calories per gram = 12 calories from protein (12 ÷ 152 = 8%)

Fat:

8 grams × 9 calories per gram = 72 calories from fat (72 ÷ 152 = 47%)

1 serving of microwave popping corn = 152 calories (45% carbohydrates, 8% proteins, and 47% fat)

---

such as carbohydrates, fats, and proteins provide energy for the body. Protein's major function, however, is to build and repair tissue rather than be used as a major source of energy. Second, protein and certain minerals, such as calcium, are nutrients that help build and maintain body tissue. Finally, nutrients such as protein, vitamins, minerals, and water help regulate body functions; for example, oxygen attaches to the iron molecules of hemoglobin and is carried to the body's cells.

Carbohydrates

Carbohydrates contribute to about half of the body's energy needs, without which no other metabolic activity could occur. They do so in the form of **glucose,** a sugar into which all carbohydrates eventually break down. In fact, glucose is the most important sugar for the cells of the human body.

There are two major types of carbohydrates. The first is called **complex carbohydrates.** They are made up of starches, the form of nutrients easiest for the body to digest, absorb, and utilize. Because of this, starches are the staple food for most of the world. Foods such as pasta, rice, whole grain breads, cereals, and starchy vegetables, such as corn, potatoes, and winter squash provide rich sources of carbohydrates. Besides providing long-term, or sustained, energy, these complex carbohydrates also supply the body with other desirable nutrients, including water, protein, fiber, vitamins, and minerals.

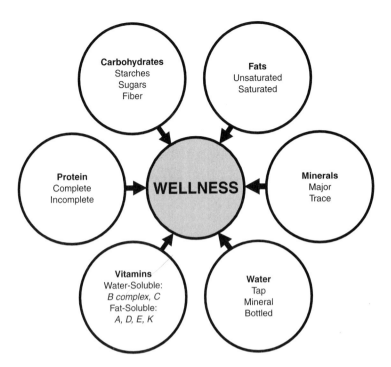

Figure 9.2
The six classes of nutrients needed for wellness.

The second type of carbohydrate is labeled **simple** because of its molecular structure. These are the sugars, which also provide energy to the body, but for a shorter period of time than do the starches. In fact, all carbohydrates, simple and complex, are changed into glucose before being used as energy by the body. Other sugars in our diet include **fructose** (found in fruits, honey, and maple syrup), **sucrose** (table sugar), and **lactose** (milk sugar).

Fiber, a carbohydrate, is associated with many health benefits even though it contains no calories or energy for the body. Known also as roughage and bulk, fiber is made up of indigestible carbohydrates that pass through the digestive tract without being absorbed. We are not able to digest fiber because the body lacks an enzyme to break it down. Table 9.2 highlights the two types of fiber, along with their sources and possible health benefits.

With a well-balanced diet, you are likely to get the different types of fiber and all their benefits. To consume enough fiber to enhance your health (25–35 grams daily), eat a well-balanced diet, making sure you consume ample amounts of whole grains, fruits, and vegetables daily. Some benefits from a high-fiber diet may actually come from the food containing the fiber, not from the fiber alone. Thus, it is better to receive fiber from foods rather than from supplements. To prevent intestinal problems such as bloating and gas, experts recommend increasing fiber gradually in the diet while drinking plenty of water.

Table 9.2   Possible Health Benefits of Fiber

Fiber Type	Source	Possible Benefits
Insoluble	Brown rice	Promotes regularity
	Dried beans	Protects against colon cancer
	Fruits	Prevents obesity by replacing dietary fat
	Popcorn	Manages blood sugar
	Rye	
	Seeds	
	Vegetables	
	Wheat bran	
	Whole grains	
Soluble	Barley	Lowers blood cholesterol
	Dried beans	Manages blood sugar
	Fruits	Prevents obesity by replacing dietary fat
	Oat bran	
	Oatmeal	
	Rye	
	Seeds	
	Vegetables	

Fats

A small amount of fat is required for good health. Fats (also known as **lipids**) provide energy, carry the fat-soluble vitamins A, D, E, and K in the blood, provide essential fatty acids needed for growth, insulate the body, are essential parts of every cell, and contribute to hormone synthesis and the blood-clotting mechanism. Unfortunately, people of all ages take in too much fat, leading to serious health problems. Health experts recommend that people, especially those at risk for heart disease, eat less fat. It is recommended that **no more than 30 percent** of your calories should come from fat, of which no more than **10 percent** come from saturated fat choices (i.e., meats, milk, and milk products).

There are two types of fats in foods—saturated and unsaturated. **Saturated fats,** except for the tropical oils, come from animal sources and are usually solid at room temperature. It is this type of fat that is associated with heart disease and cancer of the breast, colon, and prostate. Saturated fats are found in meats, butter, milk, and in the tropical oils: palm, palm kernel, and coconut.

Unsaturated fats are found in plant sources and are liquid at room temperature. Two classes of unsaturated fats are **polyunsaturated** (corn, safflower, sesame, soybean, sunflower, and cottonseed oils) and **monounsaturated** (olive, peanut, and canola oils). Recent research shows that polyunsaturated fats may also be unhealthy because they lower the "good" **high density lipoproteins (HDL)** cholesterol and may increase risk for certain types of cancer. This leaves monosaturated oils as the fat of choice. They have been shown to lower the "bad" **low density lipoproteins (LDL)** cholesterol but maintain the HDL cholesterol levels.

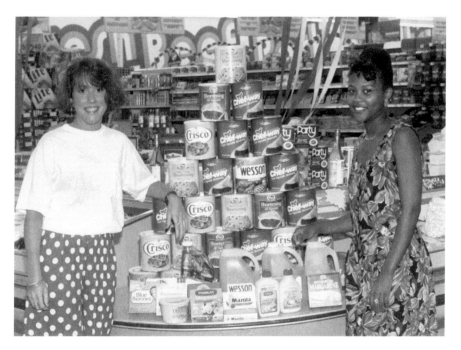

The average American adult consumes 115 pounds of fat per year.

Cholesterol is a waxy, fat-like substance that is essential for life. Cholesterol is used to form cell membranes, the sex hormones estrogen and progesterone, and other vital substances. Cholesterol also ensures proper functioning of the nervous system. It is not a required nutrient because the body manufactures all the cholesterol it needs. Excess dietary cholesterol is linked to heart disease and strokes. Cholesterol is found in all animal foods, including meat, eggs, fish, poultry, and dairy products.

Cholesterol is carried in the bloodstream by LDLs and HDLs. The LDLs are believed to deposit cholesterol on artery walls, potentially causing coronary heart disease. HDLs are thought to carry cholesterol away from the cells in the arteries and transport it back to the liver for processing or removal.

Other studies have shown that the most significant factor in food that affects blood cholesterol is saturated fat in the diet, rather than dietary cholesterol. It has been shown that when saturated fat is introduced into the body (via diet), the liver produces cholesterol, thus raising both fat and cholesterol in the blood. These studies suggest reducing total fat in the diet and exercising to lower risk of heart disease (see table 9.3).

About half of all adults have cholesterol levels that are too high. An estimated 25 percent of all Americans have high cholesterol and another 25 percent are borderline-high. Have you had your blood cholesterol levels checked recently? If not, make an appointment with your physician. Ask to receive a complete "lipid profile," which includes total cholesterol, LDL, HDL, a ratio of total cholesterol to HDL, and triglycerides.

Table 9.3 Strategies for Reducing Dietary Fat

1. Consume more grains, vegetables, and fruits.
2. Stick to recommended servings for meats (2–3 servings daily).
3. Substitute skim milk for whole milk.
4. Remove chicken skin before cooking or eating.
5. Substitute low-fat yogurt or sherbet for ice cream.
6. Purchase only lean meat cuts and trim visible fats.
7. Grill, bake, or broil instead of frying.
8. Use egg whites and limit egg yolks.
9. Limit salad dressing.
10. Limit high-fat snacks and desserts.
11. Have meatless meals once or twice a week.

Protein

Protein is needed for growth, repair, and maintenance of all body cells. Protein also transmits hereditary characteristics and helps form the hormones and enzymes used to regulate body processes. Protein can be found in animal sources (meat, eggs, fish, and dairy products) and plant sources (dried beans and peas, whole grains, pasta, rice, and seeds).

Protein is made up of twenty different amino acids. It is essential that nine of the amino acids be included in your diet, because your body cannot produce them. These nine essential amino acids must be present during the same meal in order for growth and repair of tissue to occur. The other eleven amino acids will be produced by the body. All twenty amino acids must be present in your body at the same time to form protein.

The two types of protein are called complete and incomplete. Complete protein comes from animal sources and contains all nine of the essential amino acids. One way to get all the amino acids you need is to include foods from animal sources in your daily diet. Incomplete protein comes from plant foods (vegetables and grains) and lacks one or more of the essential amino acids. If you do not eat meat products, you can still form complete protein by combining plant proteins with each other or with animal protein. Common examples of combining proteins include cereal and milk, rice and beans, macaroni and cheese, and peanut butter and jelly on whole wheat bread.

Most Americans take in more protein than necessary for good health. Your daily protein requirements are 0.8 grams per kilogram (2.2 pounds) of body weight. This amounts to no more than 12 to 15 percent of your total daily calories. A simple way to get a rough estimate of your protein needs is to take your weight and divide by three. If you weigh 150 pounds, your approximate daily protein needs would be 50 grams.

Vitamins

Vitamins are organic substances needed by the body in trace amounts. Vitamins work by enhancing the action of enzymes in the body. This enables us to use other nutrients. There are thirteen known vitamins, each responsible for performing a variety of specific and unique roles within the body. Vitamins help regulate important bodily functions such as manufacturing healthy blood cells and liberating energy from carbohydrates, fats, and proteins.

The two types of vitamins are water-soluble and fat-soluble. The vitamin B-complex and vitamin C can be dissolved in water (water-soluble) and are more readily eliminated from the body. Vitamins A, D, E, and K are transported, absorbed, and stored with body fat (fat-soluble). Since fat-soluble vitamins are not quickly eliminated, excessive amounts can lead to toxic, health-threatening effects. It should be noted that recent research has shown that megadosing with certain water-soluble vitamins has also resulted in side effects.

Most people do not need vitamin supplements. By eating a well-balanced and varied diet, you are likely to receive all the vitamins your body needs. In addition, many of our foods have been enriched and fortified, thus eliminating the need for vitamin supplementation. If you decide to take a vitamin supplement, choose a multiple vitamin that does not exceed 100 percent of the RDA. Anything above the RDA is a waste of money. In addition, there is no need to take the supplement every day because you are receiving vitamins from the food you eat. You may want to take the multiple vitamin every second or third day.

Certain people can benefit from taking vitamin supplements. Vegetarians, pregnant or breast-feeding women, women with excessive menstrual bleeding, strict dieters, and those not following a well-balanced diet should check with their physician about vitamin and mineral supplementation. In addition, those suffering from long-term illness and disease or taking medication that reduces appetite or hinders the body's ability to use nutrients should consult with their physicians.

Folic acid, a B-vitamin, has become increasingly important in our diet to help prevent birth defects along with heart disease and stroke. Research has documented the importance for all women of childbearing age and those individuals with risk factors for health disease and stroke to consume 400 micrograms of folic acid (the Recommended Dietary Allowance) every day either through diet or supplementation. Because of its increasing importance, the FDA is considering adding folic acid to flour. This, in turn, would fortify such products as breads, pasta, and cereals. In the meantime, consume foods from table 9.4 or consider supplementation.

The Antioxidant Supplement Debate

The antioxidants of vitamin C, vitamin E, and beta carotene have developed a reputation for their ability to protect us against our natural oxidative processes and ravages of the environment. Due to breathing and the normal oxidation of our cells, the body constantly produces reactive chemicals called **free radicals.** During vigorous exercise, the rate of production for free radicals increases and the body also acquires them from environmental sources such as cigarette smoke and air pollution. What is the problem with free radicals? They are unstable and wreck havoc on our stable cells. The damage caused by free radicals is believed to contribute to such conditions as heart disease, cancer, and aging. Antioxidants may protect the body from this damage by neutralizing the free radicals. Numerous studies have

Table 9.4 Good Sources of Folic Acid

Food	Folic Acid (micrograms)
Total cereal (¾ cup)	400
Lentils (½ cup, cooked)	179
Pinto Beans (½ cup, cooked)	145
Chickpeas (½ cup, cooked)	145
Spinach (½ cup, cooked)	131
Kidney Beans (½ cup, cooked)	115
Orange juice (1 cup, from concentrate)	109
Spinach (1 cup, raw)	109
Most breakfast cereals (1 cup)	100
Romaine lettuce (1 cup, shredded)	76
Split peas (½ cup, cooked)	64
Broccoli (½ cup, cooked)	39

Source: USDA Handbook 8

indicated that people who consume a diet high in antioxidant fruits and vegetables are less likely to develop diseases related to free radicals.

The jury is still out on supplements. Conflicting study results have led some to abandon antioxidants because they can often act as pro-oxidants in supplements, boosting oxidant and free-radical production. Others, notably Dr. Kenneth Cooper, the highly respected father of the aerobics movement, claim we need them more than ever, especially if we enjoy vigorous exercise. While further research is needed, it is safe to suggest that you should eat plenty of antioxidant-rich foods (see table 9.5). If you still feel you are not getting enough antioxidants from food, take a supplement, but do so in moderation.

Minerals

Minerals perform many vital functions in the body. From building strong bones and teeth (calcium) to forming hemoglobin in red blood cells (iron), minerals are essential for good nutrition. Like vitamins, minerals are needed in small amounts and do not supply energy. Other important functions include assisting in nerve transmission and muscle contraction, and regulating fluid levels and the acid-base balance of the body. Minerals can also be toxic in excess amounts. In the adult diet, mineral concerns include too much sodium and, for women, too little iron and calcium.

Minerals are classified into two types: major and trace. Calcium, sodium, phosphorous, chloride, potassium, and magnesium are considered major minerals because they are needed in amounts greater than 100 milligrams per day. Trace minerals such as iron, zinc, iodine, selenium, and copper are needed only in tiny amounts. Because minerals are absorbed, utilized, and eliminated by the body, it is important to replace them on a daily basis. Eating a wide variety of nutritious foods is the best way to obtain sufficient quantities of the essential minerals. Fruits and vegetables are ideal mineral sources.

Table 9.5   Selected Foods That Contain Antioxidants

Vitamin C	Vitamin E	Carotenoids (Beta-Carotene)	Mixed Antioxidants
Cabbage	Almonds	Apricots	Bran wheat
Cauliflower	Chick peas	Broccoli	Cloves
Grapefruit	Eggs	Cantaloupe	Green tea
Oranges	Hazelnuts	Carrots	Nutmeg
Peppers	Oatmeal	Kale	Pepper
Potatoes	Rye flour	Mustard greens	Rice
Raspberries	Soybeans	Spinach	Sesame
Strawberries	Sunflower seeds	Sweet potatoes	Thyme
Tangerines	Wheat germ	Winter squash	

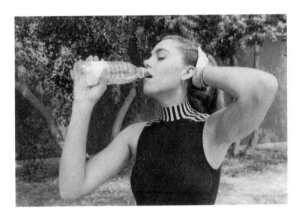

For good health drink plenty of water.

Water

Water is often called the "forgotten nutrient." Water may well be our most important nutrient because without it we would not live more than a week. More than half our body weight comes from water. Water provides the medium for nutrient and waste transportation and plays a vital role in nearly all biochemical reactions in the body. People seldom think about the importance of an adequate daily intake of water.

Adults require eight glasses of water a day, and even more with an active lifestyle. If you eat more fresh fruits and vegetables, you will require less water. Three sound recommendations for drinking more water include keeping a container of water in the refrigerator, drinking water throughout the day, and drinking water instead of beverages when dining out. Good choices are plain water from the tap and any kind of mineral water or bottled water. Many people put lemon or lime in their water to give it added flavor. Sweetened drinks (fruit drinks, soda), coffee, tea, and alcohol should be limited. Caffeine and alcohol increase dehydration and necessitate an increase in water intake.

Food Guide Pyramid

The U.S. Departments of Agriculture and Health and Human Services have adopted the Food Guide Pyramid, which replaces the Basic Four Food Groups. The new Food Guide Pyramid can help you choose the recommended servings from healthy foods to get the nutrients you need without excess calories, fats, cholesterol, sugar, or sodium.

The Food Guide Pyramid provides a simple, practical guide for general meal planning and can be used to evaluate your overall food intake pattern. The pyramid illustrates the five food groups with recommended servings that are important to a healthy diet (see figure 9.3). The new diagram places the bread, cereal, rice, and pasta group at the base, taking up the largest section. Because it is rich in complex carbohydrates this group serves as the foundation of the diet. Vegetables and fruits are two equal groups instead of one and have the next largest sections. Above them as the pyramid narrows, meats and dairy products share a band. At the top are fats, oils, and sweets, which are considered a food category rather than a food group. This category is the smallest and should provide the fewest calories.

Dietary Guidelines for Americans

The U.S. Departments of Agriculture and Health and Human Services have issued a report stating the revised set of dietary guidelines that promote realistically attainable health and dietary goals. The new guidelines promote moderation and include eating a wide variety of foods, balancing the foods we eat with physical activity, and using good judgment in our use of sugar, salt, and alcohol.

In the report, vegetarian diets were given attention for the first time. It stated that a good diet can exclude animal products like meat and milk but encouraged vegetarians to take Vitamin B-12 supplements and to find good sources of Vitamin D and calcium. Also, the report recognized recent scientific discoveries, such as the health benefit of moderate alcohol consumption and a pregnant woman's need for folic acid in her diet. The following are the new National Health and Nutritional Guidelines:

1. **Varied Diet:** Eat grains, vegetables, fruit; choose a diet low in fats and cholesterol; and watch intake of salt, sodium and sugar
2. **Exercise:** 30 minutes or more of moderate exercise most days of the week
3. **Weight Maintenance:** Weight should fall within a given range according to height (see chapter 10, table 10.1); weight loss should occur gradually
4. **Alcohol:** Drink in moderation, with meals, and when consumption does not put you or others at risk.

The 80/20 Rule

Another guide to follow for healthy nutrition is the 80/20 rule. The 80/20 rule states that if you eat a variety of nutritious foods 80 percent of the time, you can eat whatever you want for the remaining 20 percent and not feel guilty. If your diet

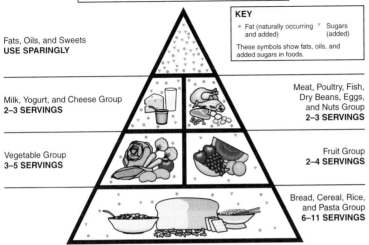

A Guide to Daily Food Choices

Fats, Oils, and Sweets
USE SPARINGLY

KEY
• Fat (naturally occurring ▼ Sugars
and added) (added)
These symbols show fats, oils, and
added sugars in foods.

Milk, Yogurt, and Cheese Group
2–3 SERVINGS

Meat, Poultry, Fish,
Dry Beans, Eggs,
and Nuts Group
2–3 SERVINGS

Vegetable Group
3–5 SERVINGS

Fruit Group
2–4 SERVINGS

Bread, Cereal, Rice,
and Pasta Group
6–11 SERVINGS

Source: U.S. Department of Agriculture/U.S. Department of Health and Human Services.

How to Use the Daily Food Guide
What Counts as One Serving?

Breads, Cereals, Rice, and Pasta
1 slice of bread
½ cup of cooked rice or pasta
½ cup of cooked cereal
1 ounce of ready-to-eat cereal

Vegetables
½ cup of chopped raw or cooked vegetables
1 cup of leafy raw vegetables

Fruits
1 piece of fruit or melon wedge
¾ cup of juice
½ cup of canned fruit
¼cup of dried fruit

Source: FDA Consumer, June 1993.

Milk, Yogurt, and Cheese
1 cup of milk or yogurt
1½ to 2 ounces of cheese

Meat, Poultry, Fish, Dry Beans, Eggs, and Nuts
2½ to 3 ounces of cooked lean meat, poultry, or fish
Count ½ cup of cooked beans, or 1 egg, or
2 tablespoons of peanut butter as 1 ounce of lean
meat (about ⅓ serving)

Fats, Oils, and Sweets
Limit calories from these, especially if you need
to lose weight

The amount you eat may be more than one serving.
For example, a dinner portion of spaghetti would
count as two or three servings of pasta.

Figure 9.3
Food guide pyramid

is consistently nutritious, an occasional hot dog or milk shake isn't going to adversely affect you. Unfortunately, too many people follow the 20/80 rule. Those who follow the 20/80 rule have diets high in calories, fat, saturated fat, cholesterol, sugar, and sodium, and low in grains, fruits, and vegetables. Knowing their diet is low in nutrients, some people compensate by adding vitamins, fiber, and an occasional bean sprout. Though it is wise to consider your nutritional needs carefully, it is not wise to lean on a magic bullet vitamin to rescue an out-of-balance diet. What kind of eater are you? Are you more likely to follow the 80/20 rule, the 20/80 rule, or some other rule?

Fast Foods

For many people, especially college students, fast foods have become a way of life. The nutritional value of fast foods, from cheeseburgers to leanburgers, can vary greatly. Breakfast foods, potatoes, whole wheat breads, salad bars, low-fat meat and milk products, low-calorie foods, and vegetable oils are examples of how fast-food companies have expanded their offerings and made foods more nutritious. Nonetheless, one glance at the menu still finds the majority of fast foods high in calories, fat, saturated fat, cholesterol, sodium, and sugar. Frying foods such as french fries and chicken breasts in oil is one reason for the high level of fat in fast foods.

Many fast-food chains now provide nutritional information for their customers. This information can keep you abreast of your nutrient intake, thereby preventing you from exceeding any maximum levels. Although fast foods can be nutritious, it would be unhealthy and expensive to rely on these foods as your main source of nutrition. **Once again, moderation is the key.**

Food Labels

Reading food labels is the best way to judge the contributions of individual foods to your daily diet and health goals. Many shoppers compare prices, but few compare labels before selecting foods. In the past, food labels have been confusing and misleading. New regulations by the Food and Drug Administration (FDA) have strict rules governing labels and descriptive terms (see figure 9.4 and table 9.6).

**Refer to Activity 9a
in the back of this book.**

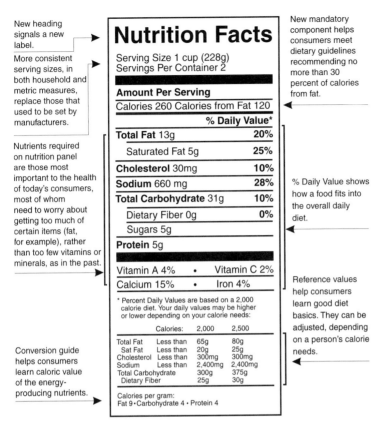

New heading signals a new label.

More consistent serving sizes, in both household and metric measures, replace those that used to be set by manufacturers.

Nutrients required on nutrition panel are those most important to the health of today's consumers, most of whom need to worry about getting too much of certain items (fat, for example), rather than too few vitamins or minerals, as in the past.

Conversion guide helps consumers learn caloric value of the energy-producing nutrients.

New mandatory component helps consumers meet dietary guidelines recommending no more than 30 percent of calories from fat.

% Daily Value shows how a food fits into the overall daily diet.

Reference values help consumers learn good diet basics. They can be adjusted, depending on a person's calorie needs.

Nutrition Facts

Serving Size 1 cup (228g)
Servings Per Container 2

Amount Per Serving

Calories 260 Calories from Fat 120

% Daily Value*

Total Fat 13g	**20%**
Saturated Fat 5g	**25%**
Cholesterol 30mg	**10%**
Sodium 660 mg	**28%**
Total Carbohydrate 31g	**10%**
Dietary Fiber 0g	**0%**
Sugars 5g	
Protein 5g	

Vitamin A 4% • Vitamin C 2%
Calcium 15% • Iron 4%

* Percent Daily Values are based on a 2,000 calorie diet. Your daily values may be higher or lower depending on your calorie needs:

	Calories:	2,000	2,500
Total Fat	Less than	65g	80g
Sat Fat	Less than	20g	25g
Cholesterol	Less than	300mg	300mg
Sodium	Less than	2,400mg	2,400mg
Total Carbohydrate		300g	375g
Dietary Fiber		25g	30g

Calories per gram:
Fat 9 • Carbohydrate 4 • Protein 4

Note: The new labeling rules won't apply to fresh meat, poultry, and fish, fresh fruits and vegetables, and restaurant food. Thus, restaurants will, for instance, still be able to use terms like "low-fat" any way they like, though consumer groups are fighting this exemption.

Figure 9.4
Nutrition Facts—Macaroni and Cheese.

Table 9.6 New FDA Regulations for Nutrition Labeling

Descriptive Term	Definition
Calorie free	Less than 5 calories per serving
Low calorie	Nor more than 40 calories per serving and no more than 0.4 calories per gram
Sugar free	Less than 0.5 grams per serving
Sodium/salt free	Less than 5 milligrams per serving
Very low sodium	Less than 35 milligrams per serving
Low sodium	Less than 140 milligrams per serving
Lite/light/lightly	⅓ fewer calories or less fat, salt, sodium, or breading than a similar product
Fat free	Less than 0.5 grams per serving
Low fat	3 grams or less per serving
Low saturated fat	1 gram or less of saturated fat per serving, not more than 15% of total calories
Leaner/lower fat/less fat	At least 25% reduction in fat or an increase in lean content in a suitable comparison
Percent fat free	Based on percent of fat by total weight—refers to portion of the product that is not fat (lean)
Cholesterol free/no cholesterol	Less than 2 milligrams per serving
Low cholesterol	Less than 21 milligrams per 3.5 ounces (100 grams)
Reduced cholesterol	At least 75% less cholesterol per serving than original product
Source of dietary fiber	10 to 19 percent of Daily Reference Values of fiber
High source of dietary fiber	20 percent or more of Daily Reference Values of fiber

Strategies for Lifetime Weight and Fat Control

10

Desire + knowledge + skills = your formula for success for lifetime weight and fat control!

Introduction

Americans spend 33 billion dollars a year on diet books, diet drinks, diet meals, and weight loss programs, according to a new study by the Institute of Medicine. In spite of spending all this money, Americans are being swallowed up in an epidemic of obesity, getting fatter and fatter. In fact, overweight Americans aged 20 to 74 increased from 1 out of 4 to 1 out of 3 between 1980 and 1990. The study also found that while more than 44 million Americans are trying to lose weight, the majority can't keep it off for more than two years. At the other extreme, the incidence of anorexia and bulimia is also on the rise. These facts demonstrate the complexity of food intake and Americans' preoccupation with their bodies.

Overweight

Many people use charts to determine desirable weight (see table 10.1). A height and weight chart can provide you with some information about how you compare to population averages. It can also give a general idea about whether you have accumulated too much or too little body weight. For excess weight, medical professionals often use 20 percent above ideal weight as an indicator of obesity. However, this method is not as accurate as measuring percent body fat because the extra weight could be composed of muscle tissue.

Although height and weight charts can serve as useful guides to maintaining desirable weight, they are unreliable as measurements for good health. Since height and weight charts represent population averages, they do not provide ideal body weight. As the population has become fatter, the averages on height and weight charts have increased. The adjustments on the charts allow individuals to have more weight and still be considered in the desirable range. Height and weight charts also do not detect levels of percent body fat—a more reliable indicator of good health than pounds on a scale.

Table 10.1   Recommended Body Weight Chart

Height	19–34 Years	35 Years and Over	Height	19–34 Years	35 Years and Over
5'0"	97–128	108–138	5'10"	132–174	146–188
5'1"	101–132	111–143	5'11"	136–179	151–194
5'2"	104–137	115–148	6'0"	140–184	155–199
5'3"	107–141	119–152	6'1"	144–189	159–205
5'4"	111–146	122–157	6'2"	148–195	164–210
5'5"	114–150	126–162	6'3"	152–200	168–216
5'6"	118–155	130–167	6'4"	156–205	173–222
5'7"	121–160	134–172	6'5"	160–211	177–228
5'8"	125–164	138–178	6'6"	164–216	182–234
5'9"	129–169	142–183			

The higher weights generally apply to men, who tend to have more muscle and bone; the lower weights more often apply to women.

Source: *Dietary Guidelines for Americans.* Washington, DC: U.S. Department of Agriculture and Department of Health and Human Services, 1990.

Percent Body Fat

The percentage of total body weight that is stored body fat is called **percent body fat.** On the other hand, **lean body weight** is the portion of total body weight that is composed of lean tissue, which includes muscles, tendons, bones, etc. It is a misconception that all body fat is unhealthy, because we each need some stored body fat known as **essential fat.** This level is the minimum amount of body fat needed for good health. Essential fat is required for such important functions as shock absorption for the internal organs, temperature regulation, and transportation of the fat-soluble vitamins A, D, E, and K within the body.

While some fat is essential, an enormous health problem in our society is the number of children, adolescents, and adults who possess too much fat (see table 10.2 for the percent body fat chart).

Obesity (Overfatness)

Obesity is a condition that indicates the body has stored an excessive amount of body fat. This condition is considered a chronic, degenerative disease that kills people and costs $70 billion annually for fat-related illnesses. There is a lack of accurate data regarding the level at which stored body fat becomes a serious health problem. However, there seems to be general agreement that men with more than 25 percent body fat and women with more than 30 percent body fat should be considered obese.

Besides having high levels of body fat, *where* people store fat may increase their risk for disease. In fact, where the body fat is located may be even more unhealthy than the amount of excess body fat. An apple-shaped body that stores fat in the upper

Table 10.2   Percent Body Fat Chart

Classification	Women	Men
Essential	<8%	<5%
Just Right	11–20%	6–15%
Desirable	21–29%	16–24%
Overfat	>30%	>25%

body may be more at risk of heart disease, hypertension, strokes, and diabetes than a pear-shaped body that stores fat in the hips and thighs.

Creeping obesity is the term used for the gradual process of people accumulating too much body fat for their health. Obesity does not occur overnight. It is months and years in the making. As we age, the extra fat accumulates as we become less active and our basal metabolic rate (BMR) decreases. BMR is the amount of energy expended at rest to sustain the vital functions of the body. For an average person, creeping obesity could result in one-half to one pound of fat gain per year.

Underfatness

Too little fat can be just as dangerous as too much fat. Females with 8 percent or less and males with 5 percent or less body fat are considered underfat. Although it is important to be aware of the dangers for obesity, excessive concern for thinness can also be a problem. America's obsession for being thin has led to an increase in eating disorders such as anorexia nervosa, bulimia, and bulimarexia. Each disorder is considered a serious health problem and usually involves the severe restriction of food and/or regurgitation of food.

Why Control Weight and Body Fat?

Achieving and maintaining desirable weight and body fat is one important goal of a healthy lifestyle. A healthy body will allow you to live life to the fullest, enjoying family, school, work, and leisure time. However, an obese or too thin body can adversely affect you in all wellness components and lead to a poorer quality of life.

Many physical problems are associated with being obese. Obesity is linked with several heart disease risk factors, including high blood pressure, high cholesterol, and diabetes. Certain cancers, such as breast cancer for women and prostate and colon cancer for men, are prevalent in the obese. Strokes or kidney problems may result from high blood pressure. The obese may also suffer from back pain and degenerative joint diseases like arthritis.

Numerous mental health problems are also linked to being overfat. In America, there is a social stigma attached to being obese. The overfat are seen as unattractive, inadequate, unhealthy, undisciplined, insecure, depressed, and having poor personalities. They are also perceived as having higher anxiety levels and having

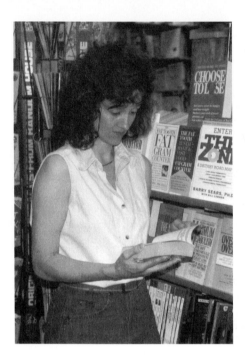

Be cautious of diet books.

lower self-concepts than normal weight people. These characteristics are certainly not true of everyone who is overfat. Those who find themselves with too much fat, however, are still perceived this way.

Also, as a result of social conditioning, the overfat often encounter teasing, ridicule, and rejection. In turn, psychological problems may result in the form of a poor body image, a sense of failure, a passive approach to life situations, and an expectation of rejection. Psychologists also think that a person may use fat as a protection from physical and, therefore, emotional relationships with others. Such a person may require therapy to lose weight/fat.

Obesity has also been linked to a shorter life span. Research has indicated that those who are moderately overfat may have a 40 percent higher risk of a shortened life span than those whose body fat levels are healthy. Also, severe obesity may result in a 70 percent higher risk of dying early that those with healthy body fat levels.

The Problems with Dieting by Itself

Study after study demonstrates that dieting alone does not work for the majority of participants. This is especially true if it is a very low-calorie diet. The multibillion-dollar diet industry wants you to believe that to lose weight and fat, you just need to follow their special diets. In fact, most diets not only fail to deliver on their guarantees, they can also lead to serious health problems such as low blood pressure, heart disease, and sudden death.

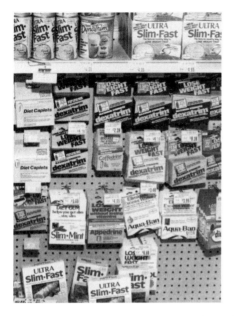
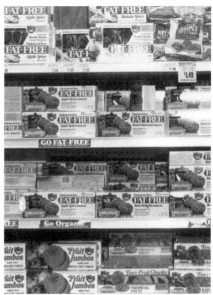

Liquid diets and diet aids can be unhealthy and seldom work in the long run.

In fact, dieting alone may slow the rate of fat loss and may predispose you to a rapid weight gain. Your body interprets dietary restrictions as famine and responds in a defensive manner by slowing its metabolic rate and enhancing its ability to store excess calories as fat. Dieting alone can also tend to use up muscle tissue, which is considered the body's fat burner. Any loss of muscle mass will lower the body's capacity to burn calories and decrease the chances of losing weight.

Analyze a diet carefully before following it. If you come across a diet that promises you the cake, icing, and candles too, evaluate it using the criteria below. Stay away from any special diets unless you get all "yes" responses from the following questions:

Does it encourage a weight loss of no more than one to two pounds a week?
Does it encourage physical activity?
Does it contain a selection of nutritious foods?
Does it emphasize medium-sized portions?
Does it use foods that are easy to locate and prepare?
Does it give you enough variety?
Can you follow it wherever you eat—at home, work, restaurants, or social events?
Is the cost reasonable?
Can you live on this diet *for the rest of your life?*

Liquid Diets and Diet Aids

Liquid diet aids can be unhealthy and seldom work in the long run. They supply between 420 and 840 calories a day, which can lead to rapid weight loss. These special diets do provide enough protein to preserve muscle tissue. However, once the dieter stops the program and returns to normal eating patterns, the weight usually returns.

Liquid diets are usually reserved for those who are at least 20 percent over their ideal weight and should only be administered by physicians. Weekly screenings for vital body functions are necessary to determine how the body is responding without solid food. Complications of these low-calorie diets include dry skin, hair loss, constipation, gum disease, sensitivity to cold, and mood swings.

Diet aids include pills such as "fen-phen"—a combination of two diet pills, the newest diet pill—Redux, diet gum, low- or no-calorie soft drinks, and low-calorie foods that may work temporarily, but are not a permanent solution.

Strategies for Lifetime Weight and Fat Control

The key to permanent fat control is a new lifestyle approach that is flexible, accepting, and family-based. It discourages calorie counting and food-focused programs that encourage dieting. The act of losing weight and fat poses certain health risks such as cardiovascular disease, high blood pressure, diabetes, and sleep apnea. Due to these potential dangers, experts strongly recommend a consultation with a physician before and during any program. This new lifestyle includes five important strategies: (1) Get Psyched! (2) Get Nutritionally Aware! (3) Change Unhealthy Behaviors! (4) Get Physically Active! and (5) Get Support!

Get Psyched!

Motivation is the drive or desire to begin or continue a behavior. It is the first step in a lifetime weight and fat control program. Your success, in large part, will be determined by your level of motivation. The more motivated you are, the better your chance of success. If you are self-motivated, you strive to reach your goals for internal rewards. Experts in goal attainment believe internal rewards such as self-esteem and self-confidence are more powerful than external rewards such as money and gifts. Whether you use one type of reward over the other, or combine both, the key is to use whatever works for you. See table 10.3 for tips on motivation.

Get Nutritionally Aware!

Since eating is one of life's pleasures, it is important to have a basic understanding of nutrition for making sensible, well-balanced food selections. The same guidelines for good nutrition can be applied to guidelines for lifetime fat control. These include eating low amounts of fat, saturated fat, cholesterol, sugar, and salt; eating high amounts of complex carbohydrates, vegetables, fruits, and fiber; and establishing healthy food relationships.

Reducing dietary fat will eliminate an enormous amount of extra calories and lead to better health. Every gram of fat you consume is equal to nine calories. This is more than double the four calories each in one gram of carbohydrate and in one

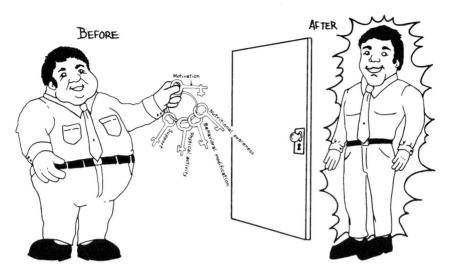

The Five Keys for Lifetime Weight and Fat Control.

Table 10.3   Motivational Tips for Weight and Fat Control

1. Think positively. Know you can and will do it. Think about the new you—feeling, looking, and functioning better, with improved health and a better quality of life.
2. Use rewards. When you reach your goals, give yourself compliments ("I did it!" and "Way to go!"). Buy something nice for yourself, too.
3. Write down at least five reasons why you want to lose weight and fat and read them daily.
4. Set realistic goals in terms of how much you expect to lose and by when you expect to lose it. Experts recommend losing no more than 1 to 2 pounds a week.
5. Visualize yourself with your new body six months from now and one year from now.
6. Write out a contract. This will raise your level of commitment.

gram of protein. Plus, the more fat in your diet, the higher your risk of heart disease and some cancers. This is true even if you are not overfat.

Follow the Food Guide Pyramid and use smaller portions. A well-balanced diet is your source of dynamic energy. When losing weight and fat, your body still needs the nutrients and calories necessary for optimal functioning. The food guide pyramid (see figure 9.3 in chapter 9) will serve as a program to follow in choosing nutritious foods. Also, smaller portions of the daily recommended servings are helpful to reduce the number of calories. See table 10.4 for additional strategies.

Change Unhealthy Behaviors!

Eating behavior is influenced by physical, emotional, and social factors. Why do you eat? Is it only when you are hungry? When do you eat? Is it only at meal times? Or when you are happy? Sad? Bored? With others? By yourself? In front

Table 10.4   Nutritional Strategies for Weight and Fat Control

1. Practice variety, balance, and moderation. Eat many different kinds of nutritious foods and use moderation for junk food.

2. Avoid diets that are less than 1,200 calories for women and 1,500 calories for men. They simply don't work for the majority who follow them.

3. Skipping meals is not recommended. After periods of hunger, metabolism slow downs and overeating may occur.

4. Be aware of the calories in foods. For example, one medium-sized apple is equal to 76 calories, whereas one slice of apple pie is equal to 345 calories.

5. If you choose to count calories, follow the 500 calorie deficit rule. Creating a deficit of 500 calories a day for seven days will equal a loss of 3,500 calories or 1 pound of stored body fat.

6. Drink large quantities of water—at least eight glasses a day. It will lower your liquid calorie intake, fill you up, boost your energy levels, and help flush out body wastes.

7. Cut out rich desserts. Enjoy nature's sweet dessert—fresh fruits. It's also a healthy way to add another serving of fruit.

8. Be warned: Grocery shopping without a list on an empty stomach is hazardous to your waistline.

9. Snack healthy: Instead of serving your body high-calorie snacks loaded with fat, sugar, and salt, serve low-calorie vegetables and fruits loaded with vitamins and minerals.

10. Think lean: Trim any visible fat from meat, remove chicken skin before cooking, and use low-fat dairy products. And go easy on the salad dressings, butter, and sour cream.

11. Remember, this is a lifetime program of good nutrition and weight/fat control. Conquer one change at a time. Then, if there is another area in need of improvement, go after it.

of the television? While you read? When you drink? When you are upset? Angry? When you celebrate? When you are depressed? Your answers may indicate that your eating patterns are dictated by factors other than hunger. Knowing why you eat and what provokes you to eat will help you improve your eating habits.

Modifying or changing your behaviors (behavior modification) is the cornerstone for a program of lifetime weight and fat control. It is built on the idea that all behaviors are learned responses from environmental cues or previous experiences. As you learn to change unhealthy habits (going back for seconds), eating becomes a more conscious act and healthy habits are adopted (eating more slowly). Table 10.5 provides examples of strategies for modifying behavior. Which ones could you employ to become a healthier eater?

Get Physically Active!

Evidence indicates that obesity is more dependent on inactivity than on overeating. Although we eat fewer calories than Americans did in the early 1900s, we are much fatter. Why? Because activity levels have declined significantly. Elevators, riding lawn mowers, power tools, remote controls, and mobile phones are just a few examples of how technology has prevented us from using more calories. Due to the sedentary American way of life, it is vital to engage in voluntary physical activity as a strategy for fat loss.

Table 10.5 Behavioral Strategies for Weight and Fat Control

1. Keep a food diary to determine eating patterns.
2. Satisfy your hunger with vegetables, fruits, and grains before eating fatty foods and sweets.
3. Slow down so that your appetite controls how much you eat. Be "in touch" with your fullness level.
4. Eat only when you are physically hungry.
5. Plan your meals in advance.
6. Concentrate only on eating. If you watch television or read while you eat, you may tend to eat more.
7. Reinforce your new healthy habits by giving yourself a pat on the back and other nice rewards.
8. Learn to relax when eating. Instead of eating when you are upset, angry, or under stress, go for a walk or listen to a relaxation tape.
9. Substitute other activities for snacking. Take a walk, read, call a friend, write a term paper, fly a kite, clean your room, etc.
10. Plan for holidays and other special occasions. If you know you are going to overeat, exercise twice that day, or lower calorie intake and exercise more the day before or the day after.
11. Use smaller plates and chew food slowly.
12. Only eat at the table. *Never* eat standing up.
13. Use self-discipline. Keep problem food (chips, sweets) out of sight and out of mind.
14. Keep nutritious food in sight and in mind.
15. Think of food as fuel for the body, instead of simply pleasure for the taste buds.
16. If you lapse (overeating, junking out) for a meal or a day, simply return to your program—think of it as a learning experience.
17. Eat breakfast. It appears that breakfast prevents hunger and subsequent overeating, reduces the amount of overall fat eaten, and helps control impulsive snacking.

The most significant factor in achieving lifetime weight and fat control is regular, moderate exercise and strength training. The American College of Sports Medicine recommends two forms of exercise for fat loss: aerobic exercise and strength-training activities like weight lifting. Aerobic activities such as walking, jogging, bicycling, swimming, dancing, and cross-country skiing are excellent calorie-burning exercises because they are performed continuously for long periods of time. Table 10.6 shows the calories expended per hour in various physical activities. Strength training or resistance exercise (weights, sit-ups, push-ups) will help increase muscle tissue, thereby increasing metabolism and using more calories.

To complement the fat-loss effects of aerobic exercise and strength training, become more active in your leisure time. To give a boost to your fat control program, you can watch less television, drive less, walk more, use stairs, plant a garden, play with the dog, and participate in active sports. The contributions of exercise to weight and fat loss are found in table 10.7.

Table 10.6 Calories Expended per Hour in Various Activities
(Performed at a Recreational Level)*

Intensity Level+		Calories Used per Hour				
	Activity	100 lbs.	120 lbs.	150 lbs.	180 lbs.	200 lbs.
Low	Pool; billiards	97	110	130	150	163
	Sailing (pleasure)	135	153	180	207	225
	Bowling	155	176	208	240	261
	Bicycling (normal speed)	157	178	210	242	263
	Social dance	174	222	264	318	348
	Archery	180	204	240	276	300
	Horseback riding	180	204	240	276	300
	Table tennis	180	204	240	276	300
	Golf (walking)	187	212	250	288	313
	Walking	204	258	318	372	426
	Baseball	210	238	280	322	350
	Softball (fast)	210	238	280	322	350
	Softball (slow)	217	246	290	334	363
	Basketball (half-court)	225	255	300	345	375
	Fencing	225	255	300	345	375
	Football	225	255	300	345	375
	Hiking	225	255	300	345	375
	Fitness calisthenics	232	263	310	357	388
	Gymnastics	232	263	310	357	388
	Judo/karate	232	263	310	357	388
	Modern dance	240	300	360	432	480
	Ballet dance	240	300	360	432	480
Moderate	Swimming (slow laps)	240	272	320	368	400
	Circuit training	247	280	330	380	413
	Badminton	255	289	340	391	425
	Ice skating	262	297	350	403	438
	Roller skating	262	297	350	403	438
	Volleyball	262	297	350	403	438
	Canoeing (4 mph)	276	344	414	504	558
	Waterskiing	306	390	468	564	636
	Backpacking (40 lb. pack)	307	348	410	472	513
	Tennis	315	357	420	483	525
	Exercise dance	315	357	420	483	525
	Weight training	352	399	470	541	558
High	Soccer	405	459	540	621	775
	Surfing	416	467	550	633	684
	Swimming (fast laps)	420	530	630	768	846
	Skiing downhill	450	510	600	690	750
	Handball	450	510	600	690	750
	Mountain climbing	450	510	600	690	750
	Racquetball	450	510	600	690	750

Table 10.6 *Continued*

Intensity Level+		Calories Used per Hour				
Activity		*100 lbs.*	*120 lbs.*	*150 lbs.*	*180 lbs.*	*200 lbs.*
Paddleball		450	510	600	690	750
Interval training		487	552	650	748	833
Jogging (5½ mph)		487	552	650	748	833
Cross-country skiing		525	595	700	805	875
Rope jumping (continuous)		525	595	700	805	875
Rowing, crew		615	697	820	943	1025
Running (10 mph)		625	765	900	1035	1125

*Note: Locate your weight to determine the calories used per hour in each of the activities shown in the table based on recreational involvement. Based on research completed at the Human Performance Laboratory, Brigham Young University.

+Note: There is no clear line of separation. Most activities are not inherently low or high intensity (except in activities like pool and bowling). How the activities are played is the deciding factor. The amount of calories burned in any activity depends on: (1) skill level of participants and (2) movement intensity.

Table 10.7 Contributions of Exercise to Weight and Fat Loss

1. **Uses Calories.** Aerobic exercise can be done at a comfortable pace for 30 to 60 minutes. With each minute of activity, you are using up more calories than you would be at rest.

2. **Increases Basal Metabolic Rate.** If you do plan to diet, exercise can help keep your BMR up when your body wants to slow it down. After finishing a workout, your metabolic rate is increased for several hours, continuing to use calories at a faster pace.

3. **Shrinks Fat Cells.** Exercise can reduce the size of the fat cells. Based on current scientific evidence, it does not appear that you can reduce the number of fat cells. However, you can shrink their size and lower your percent body fat.

4. **Prevents Loss of Muscle.** Resistant exercises such as weight training accelerate the rate of muscle buildup.

To promote long-term adherence and reduce weight and body fat, follow the FITT exercise formula. Many motivated participants, eager to lose weight and fat, start out their exercise programs incorrectly by doing too much too soon. The obvious result: another dropout statistic. Follow the exercise guidelines found in table 10.8 for a safe and effective way to reduce body fat.

At the beginning of an exercise program, a loss of inches and body fat will occur, but not necessarily weight. During the first six to eight weeks of your exercise program, you may not lose any weight. Since muscle weighs more than fat, you may actually experience a slight increase in body weight during this time period. However, because the weight gained is muscle and the weight lost is fat, you will be healthier and should experience a decrease in body circumference measurements. Beginning exercisers will often lose inches and have their clothes fit better while remaining at the same weight.

Table 10.8 Strategies for Controlling Body Fat

	Lower Limit	Upper Limit
Frequency:	3 days	7 days
Intensity:	60% of working heart rate	80% of working heart rate
Time:	30 min.	60 min.
Type:	Aerobic with strength training	Aerobic/Anaerobic with strength training

Note: Walking is an excellent aerobic activity for controlling body fat because it is low-impact, convenient, and enjoyable.

Table 10.9 Strategies for a Supportive Environment

1. Recruit at least one friend or family member who will stand by you at all times. Make out a contract and have this person sign it.
2. Announce your weight and fat control plans to as many people as possible. You will be more committed and will not want to let them down.
3. Make a game out of it. For every centimeter (ounce, inch, pound) you lose, you receive a dollar from your support team. Of course, if gains occur, you pay.
4. Stay in contact with those supporting you. Share your successes. Lean on them during difficult times.
5. Plan a celebration event for your success with your support team. Then carry it out after you reach your goals.
6. Join a support group.

Get Support!

Support from family, friends, and groups is an important piece of the weight/fat-control puzzle. No question about it—losing weight and fat is no easy task. The more ammunition you have in your arsenal, the better your chances of success. To improve your odds, enlist the support of family, friends, roommates, and groups. Maybe you can enlist a friend or family member who also wants to lose unwanted pounds and inches. Although the cheering of others can be crucial to your success, the most important support must come from you. With your personal commitment in place, your mission can be accomplished. See table 10.9 for strategies to create a supportive environment.

Relapses

Although relapses are common among participants engaging in behavior change, they can serve as learning experiences to build upon for future success. When attempting a health change, it is almost inevitable for most people to relapse and revert back to old, unhealthy habits. The three most common reasons for relapse are: (1) stress-related factors (major life changes, depression, job and school changes,

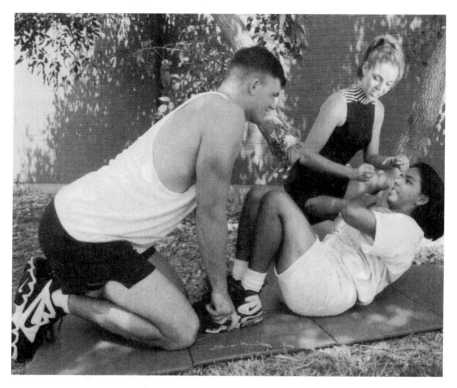

Receiving support from others is important to your weight/fat control.

and illness); (2) social factors (traveling, eating out, entertaining); and (3) self-enticing behaviors, such as putting yourself in positions to determine how much you can get away with (e.g., "one bite of ice cream won't hurt me," leading to "I'll just have one scoop," and finally, "I haven't done so well, I might as well eat the whole gallon").

Falling back to old behaviors is part of being human. If you slip back, know why and learn from the experience. Feeling guilt or anger toward yourself for not sticking with it may hinder your efforts. Just simply pick yourself up and get back on track. If you have the will, and blend it with perseverance, you will be successful with your weight and fat goals. The rewards await you.

Maintaining Desirable Weight and Fat

Once you have arrived at your desirable weight and body fat level, you are only halfway there. The challenge now is to achieve weight and fat maintenance for the rest of your life. The solution is a healthy, active lifestyle, including the five keys to lifetime weight and fat control.

Gaining Weight

Those who need to gain weight can benefit from a change in their eating and exercise patterns. Most people who desire to gain weight want to gain lean body tissue (muscle), not fat tissue. Only those who have body fat percentages below 10 percent for women and 5 percent for men will want to gain additional fat. For weight gain, consume more calories from complex carbohydrates such as pasta, rice, bread, potatoes, and cereals. In addition to a high-carbohydrate diet, regular exercise (including strength training) can add weight by increasing muscle.

**Refer to Activity 10a
in the back of this book.**

Strategies to Stay Motivated for Exercise

11

Motivational strategies—the key to staying fit all-year-round for our lifetime!

Introduction

Sticking with a physical fitness program is **exercise adherence.** Have you ever wondered why some people stick with an all-year-round physical fitness program and others do not? Is there a magic formula for being a regular exerciser? No! However, to stay with a new behavior can be a challenge, especially if you plan to be a regular exerciser after years of being inactive. This is why adopting strategies to keep you motivated to exercise is so essential. This chapter will examine strategies you can use to stick with an all-year-round fitness program for a lifetime.

Motivational Strategies

Believe in the Importance of Exercise

You must believe that there is a reason to keep exercising for you to continue doing it. A value that is based upon sound knowledge can contribute to a strong motivation to continue. If you do believe that exercise is important for you, you will likely stay with it. Those who are regular exercisers have a common belief that exercise is good for them.

Everything in life has a price. To continue any activity, you must believe that the benefits you receive from it are worth the price you will pay. To continue a regular fitness program, you must believe that the benefits you receive from it are worth your time, energy, and money.

Place Exercise As a High Priority

Regular exercise must be important enough to put into your regular schedule. If you place a high priority on your fitness program, you will fit it into your schedule. Don't let unimportant things interfere with your planned time to exercise. Make it a point to exercise at your scheduled time. Most people will respect you for sticking with your exercise commitment. Perhaps more important, you will have more respect for yourself.

```
┌─────────────────────────────────┐
│                                 │
│      Refer to Activity 11a      │
│      in the back of this book.  │
│                                 │
└─────────────────────────────────┘
```

Reach Your Goals

For some of us, the motivation to continue exercising comes from achievement. Set attainable goals for yourself. When you reach them you will feel a sense of accomplishment. Some of your exercise goals should be related to exercise adherence. One of your greatest achievements could be a lifetime of regular exercise.

Make Time for Exercise

A common excuse given for not exercising is "I don't have time to exercise." We all have the same amount of time each day, each week, each month, and each year. You must decide what is most important in your life and schedule your time accordingly. If being fit is important to you, you will find time for it.

```
┌─────────────────────────────────┐
│                                 │
│      Refer to Activity 11b      │
│      in the back of this book.  │
│                                 │
└─────────────────────────────────┘
```

Enjoy Exercise

Enjoyment is important to exercise adherence. If exercise is fun, you are more likely to do it. You can find exercise enjoyment in many ways. Some factors that bring enjoyment during exercise are selecting a fun activity, competition, excitement, relaxation, social interaction, and challenge. What produces exercise enjoyment for you?

Make Exercise Convenient

Many people claim the reason they do not exercise is because it is too inconvenient. To combat this, make your fitness program as convenient as possible. The more available exercise is to you, the more likely you are to stick with it. Here are some strategies to make exercise convenient for you: consider taking an activity class at school; locate a convenient location like your school's gym or nearby fitness center; divide your exercise into smaller blocks of time, say 15 minutes twice a day or 10 minutes three times a day; and place your exercise shoes in a highly visible place.

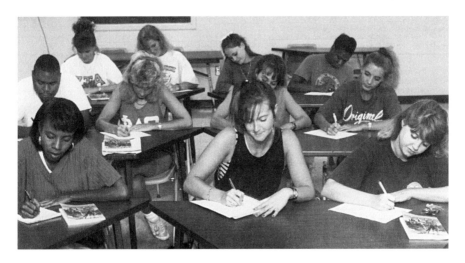

Making out a contract is a strategy for sticking with your new behavior.

Pace Yourself

If you are out of shape and want to get back in shape, take your time and pace yourself. Pushing too hard, especially when beginning a fitness program, can leave you frustrated, sore, and disinterested—exactly what you don't want! Slowly progress week by week by adding either small amounts of time, short distances, or small increases in intensity. This will help minimize soreness, bring positive results, and keep your motivation high for a lifelong fitness program.

Add Variety (Cross-Train)

Every day, there are some people who are motivated in their fitness program to do the same exercise, at the same time, and at the same intensity. Others are motivated by doing different activities, at different times, and at different intensities every day. Adding variety or cross-training could include swimming Monday, Wednesday, and Friday and weight training on Tuesday, Thursday, and Saturday. Most of us like some change in our fitness program. To stay motivated and to prevent burnout and injury, consider adding variety to your fitness program. Table 11.1 presents many popular activities you can use to stick with a lifelong fitness program.

Tell Others

If you are starting an exercise program and think you might need support to stick with it, tell everyone you know. Most of us need the aid of our family and friends to stay with our goals. Once you have told others you are going to begin exercising, it is easier to stay with it.

Table 11.1 Popular Activities and Their Important Considerations

Activity	Important Considerations
Walking, Jogging, and Running	Use quality shoes
	Walk, jog, or run facing traffic
	At night, go with other people
Weight Training	Start out slowly and progress gradually
	Consider enrolling in a weight training class
Cycling	Use a quality bicycle
	Always wear a helmet
	Pedal continuously
	Ride with traffic
Stationary Bicycling	Use a quality bicycle
	Add variety by reading a book, watching T.V., etc.
	Pedal continuously
Swimming	Improve your skill level by taking lessons
	Add different strokes for variety
	Always swim with others or make sure a lifeguard is available
Dance, Step, and Water Aerobics	Go at your own pace
	Use quality shoes
	Make sure instructor is certified
Racquet Sports (Tennis, Squash, Racquetball)	Use quality shoes and equipment
	Pace yourself when first beginning the activity
Other Sports (Basketball, Soccer, Volleyball, Golf, Bowling, etc.)	Don't overdo when first beginning the activity
	Play continuously for optimal health benefits
	Use quality shoes and equipment

Chart Your Progress

Record information about each of your exercise sessions in a consistent way. Some people use an exercise log, some use a notebook, some use a calendar, and some use a piece of paper to record their exercise accomplishments. There are many ways to do this, but somehow give yourself written credit for each exercise session.

Record information from your exercise session so you can visually see your successes accumulate. Soon you will have overwhelming evidence that you can stick with it.

Reward Yourself

Regular exercisers seem to experience a sense of satisfaction—an intrinsic reward—from regular exercise. It makes them feel good. Extrinsic rewards such as clothing,

Name_____

Walking for Fitness
Exercise Log

Day	Date	Distance	Duration	Heart rate

Figure 11.1
One example of a progress chart.

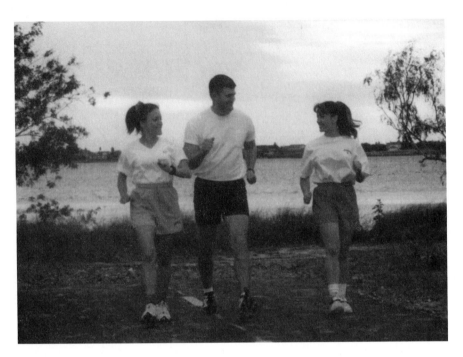

Exercise can be part of your socializing.

new shoes, and money may help get a person to start a fitness program and stay motivated for awhile. However, it is unlikely that these rewards will continue to motivate a person over a lifetime of exercise. Ultimately, if exercise does not make a person feel good, he or she will probably quit. On the other hand, people who have an intrinsic reward system and feel good about their exercise program are much more likely to stick with it.

Exercise with Others

Many people enjoy social exercise. For them, exercising with others is a powerful motivation. Some like to exercise with one friend while others like to exercise with a group. If you enjoy socializing while you exercise, build that into your plan. You may even enjoy participating in special exercise events with others, such as running or walking events. You might enjoy this for the competition, for the recognition, or for the opportunity to be with others who have similar values and beliefs about exercise.

Develop a History of Exercise Participation

As you develop a history of being a regular exerciser, it will become a part of your identity. Others will expect you to exercise. You will expect yourself to exercise.

Raise Your Skill Level

Most of us enjoy what we do well. If you are highly skilled at something, you probably enjoy it. Exercise is no exception. If you believe you are "good" at some activity, you are more likely to stick with it. To become "good" at an exercise activity, consider taking lessons. Receiving quality instruction when beginning an activity is an excellent investment of your time and money. Good lessons are generally a shortcut to better performance. Once you have learned the basic skills of an activity, it is important to continue to practice. Find partners near or at your skill level so you can both enjoy the activity together. People with similar skill levels tend to motivate each other.

Keep a Balance Sheet

Some people are motivated by a balance sheet. An exercise balance sheet contains a list of your advantages and disadvantages for exercise. The purpose of the balance sheet is to keep a focus on your reasons to exercise. Whenever you are tempted to skip a workout, look at your list of advantages. This can provide an extra incentive to put on your exercise clothes and take the hardest step of all—the first one.

**Refer to Activities 11c and 11d
in the back of this book.**

Wellness Through Healthy Lifestyles and Fitness

12

A healthy lifestyle can add life to your years and years to your life.

Introduction

> A seriously ill man went to the finest specialist in the country. After the examination, the physician presented the man with a bill for $500.
> "I can't pay this, Doc. I haven't got two nickels to my name."
> "If you haven't got any money," the doctor says, "why did you come to the finest specialist in the country?"
> "Listen," the patient replied, "when it comes to my health, money is no object."
>
> —Henny Youngman, comedian

Every day we make choices that can either enhance or detract from our present state of well-being. Although everyone desires a healthy, quality life, not everyone is willing to make the lifestyle changes necessary to bring about health improvement. However, you may be among the growing number of individuals who are striving for this richer style of life. This growth in numbers can be attributed to research findings that indicate positive lifestyle behaviors can have a significant influence on our health, quality of life, and well-being.

Wherever your health status is now, a choice of pathways lies before you. While many different paths can guide you toward better health and a richer, quality life, only *you* can choose which path to take, and at what speed you will travel. Choose wisely, and enjoy your journey.

Health and Wellness

Health is a multifaceted, dynamic quality that describes how well you are able to function at any particular point in time. Being healthy is much more than not being sick. Your health is made up of psychological, spiritual, physical, social, vocational, and environmental resources that allow you to live a satisfying and productive life. Optimal health indicates a high level of functioning and is often characterized by vitality, a zest for life, and a sense of harmony with nature and humanity.

Health is a constantly changing quality in our lives. Our health can be different from day to day and week to week due to changes in our minds, bodies, values, attitudes, beliefs, habits, and behaviors. One example of how our health can change is

Table 12.1 Major Benefits of Achieving Optimal Health

1. More "life to your years" (richer quality)
2. More "years to your life" (increased longevity)
3. A healthier mind, body, and spirit
4. Increased self-esteem and confidence
5. Greater zest for life with higher energy levels
6. More humor (fun and playfulness)
7. A positive attitude
8. Less risk for major diseases
9. Stronger immune system to ward off infections
10. More self-control and less reliance on others
11. Lower health-care costs
12. Stronger relationships
13. Improved environmental sensitivity
14. More enjoyment of your roles in life (as student, employee, etc.)
15. Better possibility of achieving your full potential in life
16. Better able to enjoy life's "moments" and experiences

depicted by Janie, a healthy, active college sophomore. Her uncertainty about what major to declare led to excessive worrying, and eventually, to a pre-ulcer condition. Once Janie declared a major in her junior year, she stopped worrying, her health improved, and she was better able to live her life to the fullest.

Wellness is a popular term referring to optimal health. Wellness includes an enjoyable and positive approach to a lifestyle that promotes a high level of well-being. It is a conscious commitment to growth and improvement in all areas of your life. The focus is on self-responsibility, self-fulfillment, and a richer quality of life. The wellness concept is based on the premise that adopting health-enhancing behaviors will help reduce potential disease risk factors and promote well-being. Table 12.1 highlights the benefits of achieving optimal health.

Health and wellness are closely related. Here is an example of how closely they work together: Having a disease (illness) is like a person walking backward; not being sick but not being well (neutral) is like a person standing still; and being generally healthy is like a person walking forward. When all your behaviors are health-enhancing, you are walking briskly toward optimal health (wellness).

The wellness-illness continuum (see figure 12.1) shows that wellness, or optimal health, is the highest level of functioning possible. The other end of the continuum represents the complete loss of functioning, or death. Where are you now? Place a dot where you stand on the continuum today. Place another dot on the continuum where you were five years ago. Which direction is your lifestyle taking you? Are your choices leading you toward a healthier and more abundant life?

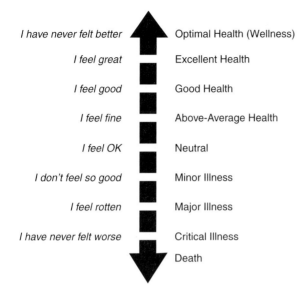

I have never felt better	Optimal Health (Wellness)
I feel great	Excellent Health
I feel good	Good Health
I feel fine	Above-Average Health
I feel OK	Neutral
I don't feel so good	Minor Illness
I feel rotten	Major Illness
I have never felt worse	Critical Illness
	Death

Figure 12.1
The wellness-illness continuum.

Health and Wellness Components

To enjoy a healthy lifestyle, many wellness components must work closely together. Your position on the wellness-illness continuum in large part depends on the daily health choices you make. It is influenced by your degree of health in each of the following wellness components: psychological, spiritual, physical, social, vocational, and environmental. The achievement of optimal health is related to being well in each of the six dimensions that follow.

Psychological

Psychological well-being combines both your emotional and mental states. It is not a static condition but a dynamic process that can change from day to day.

We all have our good days, our bad days, and our okay days. No one has total control over their emotional states (joy, sadness, fear, anger, shyness, loneliness, and guilt). However, emotionally healthy people strive to maintain psychological balance and know when to express their emotions appropriately and comfortably. They are also capable of showing respect and affection for others. In the event of emotional instability, they are willing to join a support group and/or to seek professional help.

If you have mental well-being, you can embrace reality for what it is, respond positively to life's changes, and utilize healthy coping skills to deal with stress and personal problems. Also, you believe in lifelong learning. To fulfill your intellectual needs, you keep your mind active and curious, striving to learn from all of life's experiences.

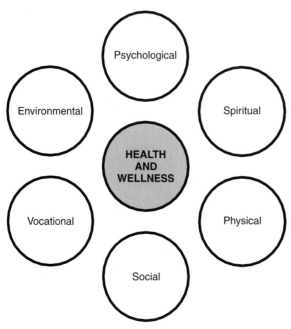

Figure 12.2
Health and wellness components.

Spiritual

Spiritual well-being is a positive sense of whatever provides meaning and purpose in your life. You can use your religion, philosophy, beliefs, values, faith, creed, principles, morals, or ethics to describe it. Knowing your purpose in life and being more comfortable expressing love, joy, peace, and fulfillment are part of spiritual well-being, which also includes helping yourself and others to achieve maximum potential.

Spiritual health also fosters a feeling of being connected with your inner self, significant others, and the universe. Finally, your spirituality includes having hope after setbacks as well as the appreciation of nature.

Physical

Physical well-being includes being physically fit, eating nutritiously, and getting adequate rest and sleep. Responsible sexual behavior and drug and alcohol use are important to this wellness component. Physical wellness includes a personal awareness and care of the physical self, which involves regular self-tests, checkups, injury and disease rehabilitation, proper use of medications, and taking the appropriate steps when illness does occur.

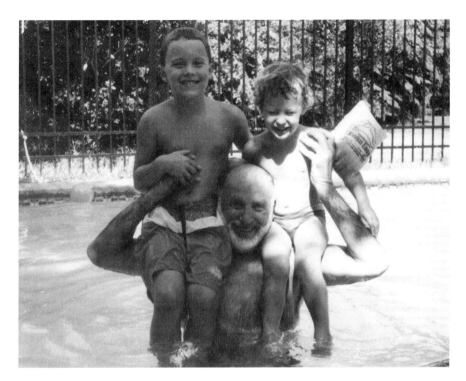

Happiness is a welcome emotion.

Social

Social well-being means having satisfying, trusting relationships and interacting well with others. It includes exhibiting fairness, justice, and concern toward and appreciation of the differences in all people. The idea of being well socially suggests having a network of family members, friends, and others who can be called upon during times of need. A socially well person also feels "connected" with their community.

Vocational

Vocational well-being is finding meaning in and satisfaction with your school, job, and leisure pursuits. Ask yourself if what you are doing right now in life is stimulating, challenging, and rewarding? If it is, you have a high level of vocational well-being. If it is not, you may want to consider making a change and seeking further training in an area of personal interest. The vocational component includes working in harmony with others to accomplish goals.

Environmental

Human survival is dependent upon air, water, and land resources. Environmental well-being refers to the impact that this natural world has on your health. It includes protecting yourself from hazards, such as secondhand smoke, which is an example of air pollution that can seriously affect your health. This component also includes being environmentally sensitive—working to preserve Earth through the four Rs: reducing, reusing, recycling, and responsibility.

**Refer to Activity 12a
in the back of this book.**

Importance of Lifestyle to Wellness

Your lifestyle (the way you live your life) plays a key role in wellness. Your health habits are the core of your lifestyle. The health choices you make will lead toward health or illness. The effects of these daily decisions are compounded over time— day by day, week by week, month by month, and year by year. The accumulation of positive choices such as fitness walking can lead you toward optimal health and a quality life. The accumulation of negative choices can lead you toward suffering, disease, and premature death.

There are other major influences besides lifestyle that influence our health. These are genetics, disease/dysfunction, access to medical care, physical environment, and psychosocial environment. Though all are critical to wellness, most health experts rank lifestyle as the most significant that you have control over. Figure 12.3 provides examples of the major influences on wellness.

Many people begin living a healthy lifestyle only after they have been diagnosed with a disease (cancer, heart disease, diabetes). Fortunately, many of these individuals are able to reverse their illness and restore their health by engaging in the positive lifestyle behavior changes ordered by their physician. Unfortunately, for many others, the damage within the body may be irreversible, leading to premature death.

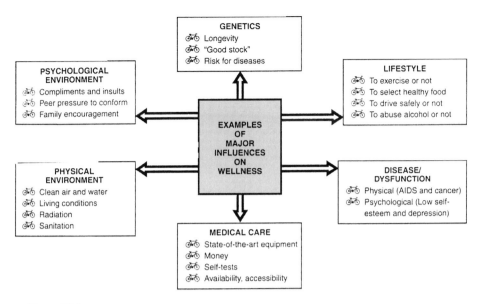

Figure 12.3
Major influences on wellness.

The Year 2000 National Health Objectives

In 1990, the health goals of the nation were outlined in the report *Healthy People 2000*. From this report, three general goals for the health of Americans were highlighted: (1) increase the span of healthy life, (2) reduce health disparities among Americans, and (3) make preventive services accessible to all Americans (see table 12.2 for selected objectives from this report).

A report card to determine progress has recently been developed for the objectives. The evaluators found that while Americans are heading in the right direction on many of the objectives, they are clearly off track in achieving others. Objectives scoring well include: more people exercising regularly and on lower-fat diets; fewer heart disease, cancer and stroke deaths; better control of high blood pressure and cholesterol levels; and increased screening for breast and cervical cancer. The objective—fewer people overweight—was one found to be headed in the wrong direction with one-third of Americans overweight. The report card indicated that instead of less Americans overweight, there are now more Americans overweight than ever before.

Strategies for Well-Being

To achieve a healthy lifestyle, consider these eight important strategies.

Table 12.2 *Healthy People 2000:* Selected Objectives of the Nation

1. Reduce overweight to a prevalence of no more than 20 percent among people aged 20 and older.
2. Reduce dietary-fat intake to an average of 30 percent or less of calories and average saturated-fat intake to less than 10 percent of calories.
3. Increase complex-carbohydrate and fiber-containing foods in the diets of adults to 5 or more daily servings for vegetables (including legumes) and fruits and 6 or more daily servings for grain products.
4. Reduce alcohol consumption by people aged 14 and older to an annual average of no more than 2 gallons per person (2.5 gallons previously).
5. Reduce to no more than 30 percent the proportion of all pregnancies that are not planned. (Since 1988, an estimated 56 percent of pregnancies were unintended, unwanted, or earlier than desired.)
6. Reduce coronary heart disease deaths to no more than 100 per 100,000 (now over 135 per 100,000).
7. Reduce the prevalence of mental disorders (exclusive of substance abuse) among adults to less than 10.7 percent (now over 12 percent).
8. Reduce homicides to no more than 7.2 percent per 100,000 (now over 8.5 percent per 100,000).
9. Reduce deaths from work-related injuries to no more than 4 per 100,000 (now more than 6 per 100,000).
10. Reverse the rise in cancer deaths to achieve a rate of no more than 130 per 100,000 (now over 133 per 100,000).
11. Reduce rape and attempted rape of women aged 12–34 to no more than 225 per 100,000 (now in excess of 400 per 100,000).
12. Increase to at least 30 percent the proportion of people aged 6 and older who engage regularly, preferably daily, in light-to-moderate physical activity for at least 30 minutes per day. (Only 22 percent of people aged 18 and older are active 30 minutes or more 5 days per week; only 12 percent are active 7 days per week.)
13. Increase to at least 20 percent the proportion of people aged 18 and older who engage in vigorous physical activity that promotes the development of cardiorespiratory fitness (now about 12 percent).
14. Reduce the proportion of college students engaging in bouts of heavy drinking of alcoholic beverages to no more than 32 percent (now over 42 percent).
15. Increase to at least 50 percent the proportion of adults with high blood pressure whose blood pressure is under control (now an estimated 26 percent for those aged 18 and older).
16. Reduce the mean serum cholesterol among adults to no more than 200 mg/dl (now over 215 mg/dl).
17. Increase to at least 20 percent the proportion of people aged 18 and older who seek professional help in coping with personal and emotional problems (now slightly over 13%).
18. Increase to at least 60 percent the use of a condom at last sexual intercourse among sexually active, unmarried women aged 15–19 (now approximately 30 percent).

1. Be Accountable

No one else is as responsible for your health as you are—not your physician, parents, friends, or partner. If you agree that health choices are mostly within your control, you will be more apt to initiate positive lifestyle changes.

2. Keep a Positive Attitude

An important strategy for well-being is to keep a positive attitude toward yourself, your health, and life in general. When you keep life positive, life has a way of keeping you positive. The following piece of prose by Charles Swindol can empower you to accept responsibility for your own attitudes throughout life:

> The longer I live, the more I realize the impact of attitude on life. Attitude to me is more important than facts. It is more important than the past, than education, than money, than circumstances, than failures, than successes, than what other people think or say or do. It is more important than appearance, giftedness, or skill. . . . The remarkable thing is we have a choice every day regarding the attitude we will embrace for that day. We cannot change our past. We cannot change the fact that people will act in a certain way. We cannot change the inevitable. The only thing we can do is play on the one string we have, and that is our attitude. I am convinced that life is 10% what happens to me and 90% how I react to it. As so it is with you . . . we are in charge of our attitudes.

3. Make Lifestyle Changes

What good is health knowledge or having positive attitudes and values if you don't apply it to life? Knowing the importance of exercise and having good intentions to be fit are admirable. However, if you don't act on this wisdom and desire, what have you accomplished? By making positive lifestyle changes, you are more likely to enjoy a high level of wellness.

4. Strive for Balance

A moderate degree of health in the six wellness components is more desirable than being strong in some and weak in others. For example, people who abuse alcohol and drugs at nightly parties may have strong social ties but are also damaging their physical health. A healthy, balanced individual can enjoy all facets of life, including school, work, family, friends, socials, and leisure time.

5. Engage in Variety

Variety is the spice of life and well-being. Staying with the same routine, physical activities, and health foods can lead to boredom and apathy. Consequently, enjoy the variety of all that life has to offer by engaging in many different activities. This type of lifestyle will promote fun and help prevent burnout.

6. Practice Moderation

Is this your belief: "Too much of a good thing is wonderful?" Any enjoyable behavior performed to excess can lead to burnout and health problems. For example, too much exercise can lead to mental fatigue and injuries. Overindulgence, even of nutritious food, can lead to excess calories and weight gain. Positive lifestyle behaviors done in moderation can keep life exciting and fun without creating unnecessary health risks. A good formula to follow is study hard, play hard, work hard—and all without overdoing any one!

7. Take Yourself and Life Lightly

Where is it written that life should always be serious and predictable? Humor (joke telling, playfulness, silliness) has been identified as the miracle drug with only funny side effects. A healthy dose of daily humor and laughter can add joy and playfulness to daily living. Physically, humor and laughter can exercise the heart muscle; improve circulation; increase alertness; and diminish tension, stress, fear, and depression. Also, a sense of humor can facilitate relationships by enhancing communication skills.

8. Have It Your Way!

It's your life and your health. Since you are the owner of your mind and body, you get to make your own health decisions. You will have your own unique wellness program tailored best to meet your health needs and interests. Once you commit to the decision that your health is a top priority, you will make everyday choices that can help prevent disease and promote well-being.

Prevention and Wellness

An ounce of prevention is worth much more than a pound of cure. Imagine you are the owner of a prized dog. To keep her healthy, you will want to give her the very best preventive care possible: lots of love and attention, the right amount of exercise and play, a special diet high in nutrients, the proper sleep and rest, and a positive, supportive environment. With this royal treatment, she is sure to enjoy a great, long life. Well, the same can be said for you. You also deserve the very best care so that you too can enjoy all that life has to offer. Performing at your full potential can lead to greater happiness, fulfillment, and a richer quality of life.

The time to strive for a high level of wellness is now. Why? First, the earlier that health-enhancing behaviors are adopted, the easier they are to be maintained throughout life. Second, the longer a person puts off living a healthy lifestyle, the greater the risk of serious disease. For example, heart disease is America's leading cause of death. While a heart attack may actually happen in an instant, it is decades in the making. Recent data by American Heart Association researchers clearly demonstrates that underactive children will likely become overweight, underactive adults with diseased arteries. Although adolescents may have no outward signs of **cardiovascular disease** they already show unhealthy changes in their arteries. Starting in middle-age or later to live a healthy lifestyle may be too late. So, if you're ready to add *life to your years* and *years to your life* then *get after it!*

> **Refer to Activity 12b
> in the back of this book.**

Activities

Activity 1a

The purpose of this activity is to observe the popularity of fitness walking.

See how many people you can find walking for exercise. Look in your neighborhood, local parks, outdoor tracks, and other likely places.

Count the number of people you see walking for exercise during a 30-minute time period. Record the number below.

_____ Number of people I observed walking during a 30-minute period.

Were you surprised at the number of people you observed walking during the 30-minute period?   Yes   No   Explain.

Name _____   To be submitted: Yes   No

Date_____   If yes, due date _____

Class _____   Score _____

Section_____

Activity 2a

The purpose of this activity is to determine the reasons for your participation in a fitness walking program. Below, list the benefits you would like to receive from your fitness walking program. Don't evaluate them at this time; just list them as quickly as you can think of them. When you can't think of any more to list, go back and place a check next to the three benefits you most hope to achieve. Of those three, which one is the most important to you? Why?

Benefits from Fitness Walking

Check off your top three.

_____   1. _____
_____   2. _____
_____   3. _____
_____   4. _____
_____   5. _____
_____   6. _____
_____   7. _____
_____   8. _____
_____   9. _____
_____   10. _____

Which benefit is most important to you? _____
Why? _____
_____
_____
_____
_____
_____

Activity 3a

The purpose of this activity is to investigate the different types of walking shoes.

Visit a store that carries walking shoes. Observe the shoes carefully to evaluate their components. You may also want to feel the differences among walking shoes by trying on different brands.

1. Which type of shoes seem to possess the better quality parts?

2. Which shoes are the cheapest?

3. Which shoes are the most expensive?

4. Which shoes offer the most support?

5. Which shoes offer the most cushion?

6. Which shoes feel the most comfortable?

Activity 4a

The purpose of this activity is to help you determine if you are medically ready to participate in a fitness walking program. Answer each of the following questions by checking "yes" or "no".

	Yes	No
1. Are you over 35 years of age?		
2. Do you have any type of cardiovascular disease?		
3. Do you have high blood pressure?		
4. Do you ever experience chest pain?		
5. Do you ever experience breathlessness?		
6. Do you have any bone or joint problems?		
7. Do you ever feel faint or dizzy?		
8. Are you a smoker?		
9. Have you been physically inactive for the past two years?		
10. Do you have a weight problem?		
11. Do you have any medical condition that could be a problem if you started walking?		

   If you responded "yes" to any of the questions, or if you have any doubt about your health, get medical clearance from your physician before starting a fitness walking program.

---

1. Which questions, if any, did you answer "yes"?_____

2. If you did answer "yes" to any of the questions, do you have medical clearance from your physician?
   Yes   No

3. If you have any health problems, have you notified your instructor?
   Yes   No

Name _____

Date _____

Class _____

Section_____

To be submitted: Yes   No

If yes, due date _____

Score _____

Activity 5a

The purpose of this activity is for you to learn flexibility exercises that can be used as part of your fitness walking program.

Perform each of the four fitness walking stretches in chapter 5 following the general tips for stretching that are also included. Check off those you performed.

Stretch	Performed
1. Lunge and shoulder stretch	☐
2. Adductor, trunk, and shoulder stretch	☐
3. Standing quadricep stretch	☐
4. Hamstring and low back stretch	☐

1. Did you enjoy performing the four stretches for developing flexibility?
   Yes   No

2. Did you experience any pain while stretching?   Yes   No
   If your answer is "yes", where was the pain located?

3. Do you plan to include stretches before and after walking?
   Yes   No   Explain.

Name _____

Date _____

Class _____

Section_____

To be submitted: Yes   No

If yes, due date _____

Score _____

Activity 6a

The purpose of this activity is to learn how to count your pulse at the radial artery and the carotid artery.

You need to know how to count your pulse before taking the Rockport Fitness Walking Test. Read or review the section in chapter 6 that explains how to count your pulse to determine your heart rate.

Find your pulse within 5 seconds and count it for 15 seconds.

Practice three times using the radial artery and three times using the carotid artery.

To convert your pulse count to heart rate in beats per minute, multiply each 15-second count by four.

Radial

1. 15 sec. count _____ × 4 = _____.
2. 15 sec. count _____ × 4 = _____.
3. 15 sec. count _____ × 4 = _____.

Carotid

1. 15 sec. count _____ × 4 = _____.
2. 15 sec. count _____ × 4 = _____.
3. 15 sec. count _____ × 4 = _____.

Which artery did you find the easiest to count your pulse? _____

Name _____

Date _____

Class _____

Section_____

To be submitted: Yes   No

If yes, due date _____

Score _____

Activity 6b

The purpose of this activity is to determine your current fitness level using either the Rockport Fitness Walking Test or the One-Mile Walk Test. Make sure you have read the medical and safety guidelines located in chapter 4 before taking the test.

Follow the directions for the Rockport Fitness Walking Test or the One-Mile Walk Test found in chapter 6. When you finish the Walking Test, record your results. Once your results are recorded, follow the directions in chapter 6 to find your fitness category.

Age _____   Gender _____

One-mile walk time in minutes and seconds _____

Exercise heart rate, 15 second count _____ × 4 = _____ BPM (not necessary for the One-Mile Walk Test)

Fitness level _____

Name _____

Date _____

Class _____

Section_____

To be submitted: Yes   No

If yes, due date _____

Score _____

Activity 7a

The purpose of this activity is to determine your exercise heart rate range. This will help you monitor your exercise intensity.

Calculate your exercise heart rate range by subtracting your age from 220. This number is your estimated maximum heart rate. Next, multiply your maximum heart rate by .60 to know your lower limit and .90 to arrive at your upper limit. You now have an effective exercise heart rate range.

Step 1

         220
       − _____   your age
       =   maximum heart rate (MHR)

Step 2

                  your MHR
       × .60
       =   lower limit

Step 3

                  your MHR
       × .90
       =   upper limit

Example

         220
       − 20   your age
       = 200   (MHR)

                  200   your MHR
                × .60
                = 120   lower limit

                  200   your MHR
                × .90
                = 180   upper limit

your lower limit _____
your upper limit _____

your lower limit ___120___
your upper limit ___180___

Name _____

Date_____

Class _____

Section_____

To be submitted: Yes   No

If yes, due date _____

Score _____

Activity 8a

The purpose of this activity is to learn correct body alignment for fitness walking.

Assume a standing position, with correct body alignment for fitness walking. Have a partner evaluate each guideline and place a check in either the "yes" or "no" column.

Guidelines	Yes	No
Head and neck erect	_____	_____
Eyes straight ahead	_____	_____
Shoulders pulled back and relaxed	_____	_____
Back straight	_____	_____
Chest lifted up	_____	_____
Abdomen pulled in	_____	_____
Buttocks tucked in	_____	_____
Elbows down at side	_____	_____
Elbows bent at 90-degree angle	_____	_____
Palms facing inward	_____	_____
Hands in relaxed fist position	_____	_____

_____ Yes, I did meet the criteria for correct body alignment.

Activity 8b

The purpose of this activity is to emphasize the idea of landing on your heel first, as opposed to landing flat-footed or on the ball of your foot.

Read technique 2, heel contact, in chapter 8. Walk 10 steps. Have a partner check to see if you are contacting the ground with the outer edge of your heel first. Your foot should also be at approximately a 40-degree angle to the ground when your heel makes contact.

_____ Yes, I did meet the criteria for the heel contact.

Activity 8c

The purpose of this activity is to experience the heel-to-toe roll.

Read technique 3, heel-to-toe roll, in chapter 8. Walk 10 steps. Have a partner watch your heel-to-toe roll. After your heel makes contact with the ground, roll your foot forward. Keep the weight toward the outer edge of your foot. Continue to roll forward until you push off with your toes.

_____ Yes, I did meet the criteria for the heel-to-toe roll.

Activity 8d

The purpose of this activity is to emphasize the push-off.

Read technique 4, push-off, in chapter 8. Raise yourself on the toes of both feet at the same time. Repeat this five times. Next, practice the push-off by walking a short distance with an exaggerated push-off. Push all the way up on your toes before breaking contact with the ground. Have a partner watch to see if you are pushing off with your toes or picking up your foot early.

_____ Yes, I did meet the criteria for the push-off.

Activity 8e

The purpose of this activity is to focus your attention on your arm swing while fitness walking.

Read technique 5, arm swing, in chapter 8. Using proper posture and alignment, practice the arm swing in a standing position and while walking. Start slowly, and gradually increase the speed of your arms.

Have a partner check to make sure your arm swing is correct.

_____ Yes, I did meet the criteria for the arm swing.

Activity 8f

The purpose of this activity is to increase your stride length.

Read technique 6, hip movement, in chapter 8. From the ready position, take one giant step forward, extending your right leg as far forward as it will comfortably go. Hold this position for 3 seconds; then lift your right foot and move it another three to five inches forward. Hold this new position for 10 seconds. Return to the ready position and repeat the procedure with your left leg. Perform this activity five times with each leg. Practicing this will help increase your stride length.

Have a partner measure your normal walking stride from the heel of your forward foot to the toes of your back foot. Then measure your stride after allowing your hips to follow through. Remember to keep your foot in contact with the ground as long as possible. Now compare the measurements to discover the extra distance in your stride length when you include the hip movement. Place the measurements in the blanks below.

_____ Normal walking stride measurement.
_____ Measurement after allowing your hips to follow through.
_____ Difference in measurements.

Activity 8g

The purpose of this activity is to emphasize the feeling of straightening your support leg.

Read technique 7, leg vault, in chapter 8. Practice the robot walk by keeping your legs straight and using the heel-to-toe roll. Do not bend at the knee. In this exaggerated activity, you will be able to notice how each leg acts like a vaulting pole.

Next, start walking in slow motion and stop just before you finish the push-off technique. Have a partner check to make sure your push-off leg is straight. Walk at progressively faster speeds, and have your partner watch your push-off leg. Make sure there is no bend at the knee until the leg starts to swing forward during the recovery phase.

_____ Yes, I did meet the criteria for the leg vault.

Activity 8h

The purpose of this activity is to learn how to add speed to your fitness walking. This technique is especially important if you plan to increase the intensity of your workouts.

Read technique 8, the racewalk, in chapter 8. After you have warmed up properly, and have walked for several minutes, move your arms and legs faster while you walk. Begin by racewalking for short distances. For recovery, use a slower pace between these sprints. Gradually increase the distance you can racewalk as you increase your cardiovascular endurance and leg strength.

Next, count the number of racewalk steps you can take in one minute. An easy way to find your steps per minute is to count how many steps you take with your right foot in one minute and multiply by two. This is much easier than trying to count every step when you are walking at very fast speeds. The maximum effective leg speed you will probably be able to achieve with a four-foot stride is about 200 steps per minute. For most fitness walking workouts, a range of 130 to 180 steps per minute is good.

_____ Number of racewalking steps I took in one minute.

Activity 9a
Nutrition Questionnaire

The purposes of this activity are to:

1. evaluate how well you eat, and
2. determine your strengths and weaknesses for the seven dietary guidelines for healthy eating.

Answer the questions for each dietary part of the Nutrition Questionnaire by placing the appropriate points in the score column. Add your scores for each part and write them in the results section. Answer the four short-answer questions in the results section.

Part I. Eat a Variety of Foods

Do you eat a variety of healthy foods each day? For each question, give yourself 2 points if your answer is "always," 1 point if your answer is "usually," and 0 points if your answer is "seldom" or "never." Maximum possible points = 10.

Score

1. _____ I eat at least six servings every day from the breads, cereals, rice, and pasta group.
2. _____ I eat at least three servings every day from the vegetable group.
3. _____ I eat at least two servings every day from the fruit group.
4. _____ I have a minimum of two but not more than three servings each day from the milk, yogurt, and cheese group (keep the point(s) if your servings above three are low-fat).
5. _____ I have a minimum of two but not more than three servings each day from the meat, poultry, fish, dry beans, and nuts group.
   _____ Total

Part II. Maintain Healthy Weight

Are you maintaining healthy weight? If you are, give yourself 10 points. If not, give yourself 0 points. Maximum possible points = 10.

_____ Are you within your recommended weight range? See table 10.1 in chapter 10.

_____ Total

Part III. Choose a Diet Low in Fat, Saturated Fat, and Cholesterol

Is your diet low in fat, saturated fat, and cholesterol? Give yourself 1 point for every "yes" answer and 0 points for every "no" answer. Maximum possible points = 10.

1. _____ My milk, yogurt, and cheese selections are mostly nonfat or low in fat (low-fat milk rather than whole milk, mozzarella cheese rather than cheddar cheese).
2. _____ I use margarine, butter, cream, or sour cream sparingly or not at all.
3. _____ I keep my servings from the meat, poultry, fish, dry beans, eggs, and nuts group to two moderate servings each day and occasionally have meatless meals.
4. _____ Before cooking and especially before eating, I remove the skin from chicken and visible fat from meat.
5. _____ I eat more fish and chicken than beef, ham, lamb, or pork.
6. _____ In preparing or ordering beef, fish, or chicken, I prefer grilling, broiling, and baking over frying.
7. _____ I choose low-fat yogurt, sherbet, or ice milk over ice cream.
8. _____ I use as little salad dressing as possible for my salads.
9. _____ When eating fast foods, I choose low-fat products (salad and fruit bar, baked potato, water) over high-fat products (cheeseburgers, french fries, shakes).
10. _____ I limit my intake of high-fat snacks and desserts (cookies, cakes, ice cream).

_____ Total

Part IV. Choose a Diet with Plenty of Vegetables, Fruits, and Grain Products

Is your diet loaded with vegetables, fruits, and grains? For every "yes" answer, give yourself 1 point. For every "no" answer, give yourself 0 points. Maximum possible points = 10.

1. _____ I like the taste of vegetables and enjoy eating them daily.
2. _____ I like the taste of fruits and enjoy eating them daily.
3. _____ I would prefer a vegetable or fruit snack over any other snack.

4. _____ If the option were available, I would choose fruit dessert over any other dessert.
5. _____ If I realize during the evening I have not consumed the recommended daily number of vegetable (three) and fruit (two) servings, I will strive to correct the deficiency that night or the next day.
6. _____ If the option were available, I would choose a wheat or bran cereal over a presweetened cereal.
7. _____ If the option were available, I would choose whole wheat bread over white bread.
8. _____ I eat products made from a variety of grains, such as wheat, rice, and oats.
9. _____ I limit high-fat grains in my diet (croissants, cakes, cookies).
10. _____ I strive to eat a minimum of six servings each day of bread, cereal, rice, and pasta products.
_____ Total

Part V. Use Sugars Only in Moderation

What size (small, medium, large, or humongous) is your sweet tooth? For every "yes" answer to the following statements, give yourself 1 point. For every "no" answer, give yourself 0 points. Maximum possible points = 5.

1. _____ I limit sugar intake whenever possible.
2. _____ I do not like candy or chocolate.
3. _____ I would prefer cereal, tea, and coffee with no sugar or sweeteners added. (Keep the point if you don't eat cereal or drink tea or coffee.)
4. _____ I drink more water and milk than sweetened liquids such as soft drinks.
5. _____ I prefer snacks that contain no sugar, low sugar, or natural sugar (vegetables, fruits) over high-sugar snacks and desserts (cookies, cakes).
_____ Total

Part VI. Use Salt and Sodium Only in Moderation

What size mountain (small, medium, or high) of salt are you on? If your answer to each of the following statements is "always," give yourself 2 points. If your answer is "usually," give yourself 1 point, and 0 points if your answer is "seldom" or "never." Maximum possible points = 4.

1. _____ I choose foods lightly salted or not salted at all.
2. _____ I add little or no salt either while cooking foods or when eating them.
_____ Total

Part VII. If You Drink Alcoholic Beverages, Do So in Moderation

If you drink alcohol, do you drink in moderation? For every "yes" answer, give yourself 5 points. For every "no" answer, give yourself 0 points. Maximum possible points = 10.

1. _____ I do not drink more than two alcoholic beverages in a day. One drink is 5 oz. of wine, 10 oz. wine cooler, 12 oz. beer, or 1 oz. hard liquor (whiskey, gin, rum, vodka).

2. _____ Rarely or never do I skip entire meals or major portions of meals because my stomach is full from drinking alcoholic beverages.

_____ Total

Results

After totaling your scores for each part, write them on the following blanks.

Part I.	_____
Part II.	_____
Part III.	_____
Part IV.	_____
Part V.	_____
Part VI.	_____
Part VII.	_____
Total	_____ (out of 59)

59	Superior food selection
50–59	Healthy food selection
40–49	Not bad, but room for improvement
30–39	Below average. Consider eating for your health and not just your taste buds.
Below 30	Make an appointment with your instructor, your physician, or a dietitian for immediate dietary counsel.

1. Do you feel your rating accurately reflects your nutritional health? Explain.

2. In what dietary guidelines are you strong?

3. In what dietary guidelines, if any, are you weak?

4. What did you learn from this questionnaire? Will you apply this information to your daily food selections?

Activity 10a

The purpose of this activity is to design your own weight and fat control program. Whether you plan to lose, maintain, or gain weight and fat, this contract will be helpful in reaching your goals.

I, _____, commit myself to a weight and fat management

program beginning _____. I plan to _____

(lose/gain/maintain) weight and fat, using the five strategies that follow.

Motivation

Which motivational tips do you plan to follow? (See table 10.3 in chapter 10.)

1. _____
2. _____
3. _____
4. _____
5. _____

Nutritional Awareness

Which nutritional strategies do you plan to adopt in order to eat better? (See table 10.4 in chapter 10.)

1. _____
2. _____
3. _____
4. _____
5. _____

Behavior Modification

Which behavior modification tips do you plan to adopt to develop better eating behaviors? (See table 10.5 in chapter 10.)

1. _____
2. _____
3. _____
4. _____
5. _____

Physical Activity

How would you rate your current level of activity: high, medium, or low?

_____

Check these exercise guidelines you plan to follow:

Frequency	—5 to 7 days a week	_____
Intensity	—Elevate the heart rate.	_____
Time	—30 to 60 minutes	_____
Type	—Aerobic	_____
Start slowly	—Gradual build up.	_____
Strength training	—Light weights, many repetitions	_____

Which form of exercise (walking, swimming, bicycling, dancing, jogging, etc.) are

you most likely to stay with? _____

Supportive Environment

Have your support team (family, friends, and others) write their names on the following lines, signifying their support for your fat control program.

_____

_____

_____

_____

_____

_____

Name _____   To be submitted: Yes   No

Date _____   If yes, due date _____

Class _____   Score _____

Section_____

Activity 11a

The purpose of this activity is to help you set priorities and identify those things that are most important to you.

List the 10 most important things in your life right now. After you have written them down, rank them from 1 to 10 (1 being the most important).

Rank

_____ _____

_____ _____

_____ _____

_____ _____

_____ _____

_____ _____

_____ _____

_____ _____

_____ _____

_____ _____

---

1. Does fitness walking contribute to any of the 10 most important things in your life right now?
   Yes   No

2. If your answer is "yes", how high was the ranking of the item(s)?

Activity 11b

The purpose of this activity is to fill out a fitness walking contract, which will affirm your commitment to reach the goals you have set for yourself.

Once you have clearly defined your goals, fill in the contract.

I, _____, will commit myself to being in better health by following a fitness walking program.

The specific health and fitness goals of my walking program are:

1.
2.
3.

The specific date(s) I expect to reach my goal(s) is(are):

Other important reasons I have committed myself to a fitness walking program are:

1.
2.
3.

Guidelines to follow that will help me stay with my fitness walking program are:

1.
2.
3.

Support people who will help me with my fitness walking program are:

1.
2.
3.

When I reach my goals, I will reward myself by doing the following:

Signature _____ Date_____
Witness_____ Witness _____

Name _____

Date _____

Class _____

Section _____

To be submitted: Yes   No

If yes, due date _____

Score _____

Activity 11c

The purpose of this activity is to create a personal balance sheet to see the advantages and disadvantages of participating in a fitness walking program.

On the left side, list all of the benefits and advantages to be gained by regular participation in a fitness walking program. Refer to chapters 2, 9, 10, and 12 to remember the advantages and benefits of walking. When you have listed all of the advantages and benefits you can find in this book and all of the other advantages and benefits you can think of, go to the right side of the page and list the disadvantages of participating in a fitness walking program.

Post this list where you will see it every day. When you feel like skipping a workout, look at the advantages and benefits column. This will encourage you to "get going" with your workout.

Advantages and benefits	Disadvantages

Name _____

Date _____

Class _____

Section_____

To be submitted: Yes   No

If yes, due date _____

Score _____

Activity 11d

The purpose of this activity is to identify motivational strategies that will help you stick with your fitness walking program.

   Place a check by all of the motivational strategies you believe will help you stick with your fitness walking program. Once you have selected these strategies, try each one. Then incorporate into your fitness walking program the strategies that work best for you.

_____   Set clear and definite goals
_____   Maintain a positive attitude
_____   Plan
_____   Do it
_____   Reward yourself
_____   Make fitness walking a priority
_____   Create a personal balance sheet
_____   Chart your progress
_____   Walk with others
_____   Add variety
_____   Select a pleasing route
_____   Cross-train
_____   Reduce barriers to exercise
_____   Join a club
_____   Participate in special events
_____   Evaluate and modify

What strategies work best for you?

Activity 12a

The purpose of this activity is to assess your current level of wellness in the eight dimensions.

Review the eight wellness components found in chapter 12. In the Wellness Wheel on the next page, place a dot on each line that best represents where you feel you are now. Dots placed close to the inner circle (hub) represent a lower level of health, whereas dots placed near the outer circle (rim) indicate a higher level of health. Next, connect the dots.

Results

How balanced is your development? (Will your wheel roll or crash after the first turn?)

_____

_____

_____

Are you close to achieving a high level of health in each dimension? _____
What are your strengths? What are your weaknesses?

Strengths	Weaknesses
1. _____	_____
2. _____	_____
3. _____	_____
4. _____	_____
5. _____	_____
6. _____	_____
7. _____	_____
8. _____	_____

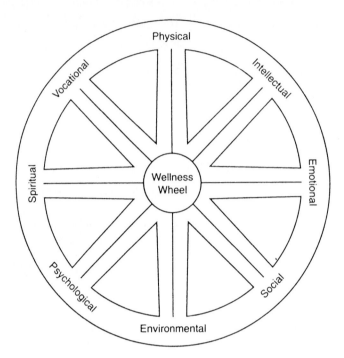

Wellness Wheel. All eight components influence your level of wellness.

What behaviors can you eliminate, modify, or adopt to improve your health?

Eliminate: _____

Modify: _____

Adopt: _____

Activity 12b

The purpose of this activity is to help you identify lifestyle behaviors that are enhancing or harming your health.

    Place a check in the positive or negative column for each lifestyle behavior. A check in the positive column indicates this behavior is either enhancing your health or not harming your health. A check in the negative column indicates this behavior may be harming your health.

    Add up the positive behaviors and the negative behaviors and place in the total column on the next page. Are you satisfied with your results? What are your healthy lifestyle behaviors? What are your unhealthy lifestyle behaviors? What are your strategies to improve the lifestyle behaviors that are taking away from your health?

Lifestyle Behavior

Do you	Yes	No
Refrain from using tobacco (including smokeless tobacco)	____	____
Avoid smoke-filled environments	____	____
Avoid use of alcohol in excess	____	____
Maintain a healthy body weight	____	____
Maintain a healthy percent of body fat	____	____
Maintain healthy blood pressure	____	____
Receive adequate amounts of sleep and rest	____	____
Maintain a regular exercise program	____	____
Practice stress management techniques	____	____
Eat breakfast	____	____
Maintain a well-balanced diet	____	____
Consume six daily servings of grains	____	____
Consume three servings of vegetables daily	____	____
Consume two servings of fruits daily	____	____
Limit salt intake	____	____
Limit sugar intake	____	____
Limit fat intake	____	____
Wear seat belts regularly	____	____
Refrain from drinking and driving	____	____
Receive regular physical examinations	____	____

Receive regular dental examinations   _____ _____
Perform monthly self-exam for lumps/thickening of the skin   _____ _____
Practice safe sex   _____ _____
Maintain positive attitude toward life   _____ _____
Avoid the use illegal drugs   _____ _____
Total   _____ _____

What do your answers tell you? _____

_____

_____

_____

Appendix A
Walking for Fitness Exercise Log

Name _____

Walking for Fitness
Exercise Log

Day	Date	Distance	Duration	Heart rate

Appendix B
Resources for Fitness Walking

Information

The Rockport Company
72 Howe St.
Marlboro, MA 01752

Periodicals

The Walking Magazine
P.O. Box 52341
Boulder, CO 80321-2341

The Atlantic Trailmaster Magazine
6904 Beech Ave.
Baltimore, MD 21206-1200

Walking! Journal
Box 454
Athens, GA 30603

Heart and Sole Newsletter
National Organization of Mall
 Walkers
P.O. Box 191
Hermann, MO 65041

WalkWays
WalkWays Center
733 15th St., NW
Washington, DC 20025

Walking Tapes

Hooked On Walking
P.O. Box 885
Cypress, TX 77429

Fitness Walking
Arena Marketing
P.O. Box 32080
Kansas City, MO 76411

Happy Walking Tapes
Happy Heart Productions Inc.
Box 1015
Ballwin, MO 63011-9998

Rhythm Walking Tapes
K-Tel
P.O. Box 46004
Minneapolis, MN 55446-9004

Music to Walk By
WalkUSA
6310 Nancy Ridge Road
Ste. 101
San Diego, CA 92121-3209

Walking Tapes
Box 767364
Roswell, GA 30076

Walking Equipment

WalkUSA
1–800–255–6422

The Sportsvilla
Box 209
Vandalia, MO 63382

PermaID
P.O. Box 400
Columbia, MD 21045

Creative Health Products, Inc.
1000 Saddle Ridge Rd.
Plymouth, MI 48170

Walking Organizations

American Volkssport Association
Suite 101
Phoenix Square 1001
Pat Booker Road
Universal City, TX 78148

Hot Line 1–800–830–WALK

National Association of Mall Walkers
P.O. Box 191
Hermann, MO 65041

International Walking Society
P.O. Box 4037
Boulder, CO 80306

Walking Association
655 Rancho Catalina Place
Tucson, AZ 86704

Walking World Institute
P.O. Box K Gracie Station
New York, NY 10028
(212) 988–8319

Walking Tours

Country Walkers
P.O. Box 180 W
Waterbury, VT 05676

Progressive Trails, Inc.
1932 1st Ave., Ste. 1100-W
Seattle, WA 98101

Distant Journeys
P.O. Box 1211
Camden, ME 04843

Roads Less Traveled
P.O. Box 18742-K3
Boulder, CO 80308

References and Suggestions for Further Reading

Allsen, P. E., Harrison, J. M., & Vance, B. (1997). *Fitness for Life: An Individualized Approach.* 7th ed. Dubuque, IA: Wm. C. Brown.

Alter, M. J. (1988). *Science of Stretching.* Champaign, IL: Human Kinetics.

Althoff, S. A., Svoboda, M., & Girdano, D. A. (1988). *Choices in Health and Fitness for Life.* Scottsdale, AZ: Gorsuch Scarisbrick.

American Cancer Society. *Cancer Facts and Figures.* Atlanta, GA: American Cancer Society, 1996.

———. *The Smoke Around You: The Risks of Involuntary Smoking.* Atlanta, GA: American Cancer Society, 1995.

———. *Taking Control: 10 Steps to a Healthier Life and Reduced Cancer Risk.* Atlanta, GA: American Cancer Society, 1992.

American College of Sports Medicine. *Guidelines for Graded Exercise Testing and Exercise Prescription.* 5th ed. Philadelphia: Lea & Febiger, 1995.

———. *The American Heart Association Diet: An Eating Plan for Healthy Americans.* Dallas, TX: American Heart Association, 1993.

———. *1996 Heart and Stroke Facts.* Dallas, TX: American Heart Association, 1995.

Anderson, B. (1980). *Stretching.* Bolinas, CA: Shelter.

Anspaugh, D. J., Hamrick, M. H., & Rosato, F. D. (1994). *Wellness: Concepts and Applications.* 2d ed. St. Louis: Mosby.

Ardell, D. B. (1985). *The History and Future of Wellness.* Dubuque, IA: Kendall/Hunt.

Ardell, D. B., & Tager, M. J. (1988). *Planning for Wellness: A Guidebook for Achieving Optimal Health.* 3d ed. Dubuque, IA: Kendall/Hunt.

Brody, J. "Walking for Fitness," *Corpus Christi (Texas) Caller Times,* 20 May 1966, pp. 6–7.

Brooks, G. A., & Fahey, T. D. (1985). *Exercise Physiology: Human Bioenergetics and Its Applications.* New York: Macmillan.

Brooks, G. A., & Fahey, T. D. (1987). *Fundamentals of Human Performance.* New York: Macmillan.

Brown, H. L. (1992). *Lifetime Fitness.* 3d ed. Scottsdale, AZ: Gorsuch Scarisbrick.

Cairns, M. (1985). Racewalking—A Fitness Alternative. *Journal of Physical Education, Recreation, and Dance,* 50–51.

Callaway, C. W. (1988). Biological Adaptations to Starvation and Semistarvation. In R. T. Frankie & M. Yang (Eds.), *Obesity and Weight Control.* Rockville, MD: Aspen.

Campbell, K. R., Adres, R., Greer, N. L., Hintermeister, R., & Rippe, J. (1987). The Effects of Fatigue on Selected Biomechanical Parameters in Fitness Walking. *Medicine and Science in Sports and Exercise,* 19, 518.

Coleman, R. J., Wilkie, S., Viscio, L., O'Hanley, S., Porcari, J., Kline, G., Keller, B., Hsieh, S., Freedson, P. S., & Rippe, J. (1987). Validation of a One-Mile Test for Estimating $\dot{V}O_2$max in 20–29 Year Olds. *Medicine and Science in Sports and Exercise,* 19, 528.

Cooper, K. H. (1968). *Aerobics.* New York: Bantam.

Cooper, K. H. (1970). *The New Aerobics.* New York: Bantam.

Cooper, K. H. (1977). *The Aerobics Way.* New York: Bantam.

Cooper, K. H. (1982). *The Aerobics Program for Total Well-Being: Exercise, Diet, Emotional Balance.* New York: Bantam.

Cooper, M., & Cooper, K. H. (1972). *Aerobics for Women.* New York: Bantam.

Corbin, C. B., & Lindsey, R. (1997). *Concepts of Physical Fitness with Laboratories.* 9th ed. Dubuque, IA: Wm. C. Brown.

Corbin, D. E. (1988). *Jogging.* Glenview, IL: Scott, Foresman.

Couey, R. B. (1982). *Building God's Temple.* Minneapolis: Burgess.

DeBenedette, V. (August 1988). Keeping Pace with the Many Forms of Walking. *The Physician and Sportsmedicine* 16(8): 145–150.

deVries, H. A. (1986). *Physiology of Exercise: For Physical Education and Athletics.* 4th ed. Dubuque, IA: Wm. C. Brown.

DiGennaro, J. (1983). *The New Fitness: Exercise for Everybody.* Englewood, CO: Morton.

Dishman, R. K. (Ed.). (1988). *Exercise Adherence: Its Impact on Public Health.* Champaign, IL: Human Kinetics.

Feeney, P. (Ed.). (1990). *What's in a Label? A Dietitian's Handbook for Helping Consumers Demystify Food Labels.* American Dietetic Association and ConAgra. Chicago, IL.

Fixx, J. F. (1977). *The Complete Book of Running.* New York: Random House.

Fox, E. L., Bowers, R. W., & Foss, M. L. (1989). *The Physiological Basis of Physical Education and Athletics.* 4th ed. Philadelphia: Saunders.

Friedman, R. M. (Ed.). (October 1988). Fatter Calories. *University of California, Berkeley Wellness Letter,* 5, 1–2.

Greenberg, J. S., & Pargman, D. (1989). *Physical Fitness: A Wellness Approach.* 2d ed. Englewood Cliffs, NJ: Prentice-Hall.

Greer, N., Campbell, K., Andres, R., Hintermeister, R., & Rippe, J. (1987). An Evaluation of Walking and Running Shoes During Walking. *Medicine and Science in Sports and Exercise,* 19, 517.

Greer, N. L., Campbell, K. R., Foley, P. M., Andres, R. O., & Rippe, J. M. (1986). An Assessment of the Reliability of Ground Reaction Forces During Walking. *Medicine and Science in Sports and Exercise,* 18, S81.

Hales, D. (1997). *An Invitation to Health.* 7th ed. Redwood City, CA: Benjamin/ Cummings.

Hawkins, J. D., & Weigle, S. M. (1997). *Walking for Fun and Fitness.* 2d ed. Englewood, CO: Morton.

Henderson, J. (1988). *Total Fitness: Training for Life.* Dubuque, IA: Wm. C. Brown.

Hesson, J. L. (1997). *Weight Training for Life.* 4th ed. Englewood, CO: Morton.

Iknoian, Therese. (1995). *Fitness Walking.* Champaign, IL: Human Kinetics.

Jonas, S., & Radetsky, P. (1988). *PaceWalking: The Balanced Way to Aerobic Health.* New York: Crown.

Kahnert, J. H. (1981). *Excellence in Physical Fitness.* 2d ed. Dubuque, IA: Kendall/Hunt.

Kashlwa, A., & Rippe, J. (1987). *Fitness Walking for Women.* New York: Putnam.

Katch, F. I., & McArdle, W. D. (1983). *Nutrition, Weight Control and Exercise.* 2d ed. Philadelphia: Lea and Febiger.

Keesey, R. E. (1986). A Set-Point Theory of Obesity. In K. D. Brownell & J. P. Foreyt (Eds.), *Handbook of Eating Disorders.* New York: Basic.

Kemper, D. K., Giuffre, J., & Drabinski, G. (1985). *Pathways: A Successful Guide for a Healthy Life.* Boise, ID: Healthwise.

Kline, G., Porcari, J., Freedson, P., Ward, A., Ross, J., Wilkie, S., & Rippe, J. (1987). Does Aerobic Capacity Affect the Validity of the One Mile Walk $\dot{V}O_2$max Prediction? *Medicine and Science in Sports and Exercise,* 19, 528.

Kline, G., Porcari, J., Hintermeister, R., Freedson, P., McCarron, R., Rippe, J., Ross, J., Ward, A., & Gurry, M. (1986). Prediction of $\dot{V}O_2$max from a One-Mile Track Walk. *Medicine and Science in Sports and Exercise,* 18, S35.

Kline, G. M., Porcari, J. P., Hintermeister, R., Freedson, P. S., Ward, A., McCarron, R. F., Ross, J., & Rippe, J. M. (1987). Prediction of $\dot{V}O_2$max from a One-Mile Track Walk. *Medicine and Science in Sports and Exercise,* 19, 253.

Koszuta, L. E. (August/September 1988). Splash On By. *The Walking Magazine,* Vol. 4, 65–70.

Kuntzleman, C. T., & Editors of Consumer Guide. (1978). *The Complete Book of Walking.* New York: Simon and Schuster.

Kusinitz, I., & Fine, M. (1991). *Your Guide to Getting Fit.* 2d ed. Palo Alto, CA: Mayfield.

Lamb, D. R. (1984). *Physiology of Exercise: Responses & Adaptations.* 2d ed. New York: Macmillan.

Levy, M. R., Dignan, M., & Shirreffs, J. H. (1992). *Life and Health: Targeting Wellness.* New York: McGraw-Hill.

Makalous, S. L., Arauj, M. A., & Thomas, T. R. (April 1988). Energy Expenditure during Walking with Hand Weights. *The Physician and Sportsmedicine,* 16(4): 139–148.

Mayer, J. (1975). *A Diet for Living.* New York: David McKay.

Mayer, J. (1975) An Hour of Exercise vs. a Pound of Flesh. In B. Q. Hafen (Ed.), *Overweight and Obesity: Causes, Fallacies,*

Treatment. Provo, UT: Brigham Young University Press.

Mazzeo, K. S. (1985). *A Commitment to Fitness*. Englewood, CO: Morton.

McArdle, W. D., Katch, F. I., & Katch, V. L. (1991). *Exercise Physiology: Energy, Nutrition, and Human Performance*. 3d ed. Philadelphia: Lea & Febiger.

McCarron, R., Kline, G., Freedson, P., Ward, A., & Rippe, J. (1986). Fast Walking Is an Adequate Aerobic Stimulus for High Fit Males. *Medicine and Science in Sports and Exercise*, 18, S21.

McGlynn, G. (1996). *Dynamics of Fitness: A Practical Approach*. 4th ed. Dubuque, IA: Wm. C. Brown.

Melograno, V. J., & Klinzing, J. E. (1988). *An Orientation to Total Fitness*. 4th ed. Dubuque, IA: Kendall/Hunt.

Miller, D. K., & Allen, T. E. (1986). *Fitness: A Lifetime Commitment*. 3d ed. Edina, MN: Burgess.

Montoye, H. J., Christian, J. L., Nagle, F. J., & Levin, S. M. (1988). *Living Fit*. Menlo Park, CA: Benjamin/Cummings.

Morrison's Custom Management. (1992). *Nutrition Choices for a Healthful Lifestyle*. Mobile, AL.

Morrison's Custom Management. (1992). *Strides for Life Walking and Nutrition Education Program*. Mobile, AL.

Nestle Worldview. (Spring 1992). *Cholesterol: The Villain Revisited*. (Vol. 4, No. 1). Washington, DC: Nestle Information Service.

Nestle Worldview. (Spring 1992). *Maintaining a Healthy Weight* (Vol. 4, No. 1). Washington, DC: Nestle Information Service.

Nestle Worldview. (Spring 1992). *Weighing the Facts on Obesity* (Vol. 4, No. 1). Washington, DC: Nestle Information Service.

Nestle Worldview. (Winter 1992) *Vitamins: Building Blocks of Better Health* (Vol. 3, No. 4). Washington, DC: Nestle Information Service.

Noble, B. J. (1986). *Physiology of Exercise and Sport*. St. Louis: Times Mirror/Mosby.

O'Hanley, S., Ward, A., Zwiren, L., McCarron, R., Ross, J., & Rippe, J. M. (1987). Validation of a One-Mile Walk Test in 70–79 Year-Olds. *Medicine and Science in Sports and Exercise*, 19, 528.

Porcari, J., Kline, G., Hintermeister, R., Freedson, P., Ward, A., Gurry, M., Ross, J., McCarron, R., & Rippe, J. (1986). Is Fast Walking an Adequate Aerobic Training Stimulus? *Medicine and Science in Sports and Exercise*, 18, S81.

Porcari, J., McCarron, R., Kline, G., Freedson, P., Ward, A., Ross, J., & Rippe, J. (1987). Is Fast Walking an Adequate Aerobic Training Stimulus in 30–69 Year Old Adults? *The Physician and Sports Medicine*, 15, 119.

Powers, Scott K. & Dodd, Scott K. *The Essentials of Total Fitness*. (1997). Needham Heights, MA: Allyn & Bacon.

Prentice, W. E. *Get Fit, Stay Fit*. 3d ed. St. Louis, MO: Mosby Year Book.

Rippe, J., Ross, J., Gurry, M., Hitzhusen, J., & Freedson, P. (July 1985). Cardiovascular Effects of Walking. *Proceedings of the Second International Conference of Physical Activity, Aging, and Sports*, p. 47.

Rippe, J., Ross, J., McCarron, R., Porcari, J., Kline, G., Ward, A., Gurry, M., & Freedson, P. (1986). One-Mile Walk Time Norms for Healthy Adults. *Medicine and Science in Sports and Exercise*, 18, S21.

Rippe, J. M., Ward, A., & Freedson, P. (1988). Walking for Health and Fitness. In *Encyclopedia Brittanica Medical and Health Annual*.

Robbins, G., Powers, D., & Burgess, S. (1997). *A Wellness Way of Life*. 3d ed. Dubuque, IA: Wm. C. Brown.

Rockport Company. (1990). *The Rockport Guide to Fitness Walking*. Marlboro, MA: Rockport Walking Institute.

Rockport Company. (1990). *Walk Leader Manual*. Marlboro, MA: Rockport Walking Institute.

Ross, J., Gurry, M., Ward, A., Walcott, G., Hitzhusen, J., & Rippe, J. (1986). Accuracy of Predicted Max Heart Rate in the Elderly. *Medicine and Science in Sports and Exercise*, 18, S95.

Schwartz, L. (1987). *Heavyhands Walking*. Emmaus, PA: Rodale.

Seiger, L. H., & Hesson, J. L. (1994). *Walking for Fitness*. Dubuque, IA: Wm. C. Brown.

Seiger, L. H. & Richter, J. (1997). *Your Health, Your Style: Strategies for Wellness*. Dubuque, IA: Wm. C. Brown.

Seiger, L. H., Vanderpool, K. & Barnes, D. (1995). *Fitness and Wellness Strategies*. Dubuque, IA: Wm. C. Brown.

Siegel, A. J. (Nov./Dec. 1988). New Insights about Obesity and Exercise. *Your Patient and Fitness in Cardiology* (Vol. 2, No. 6). McGraw-Hill, Minneapolis, MN.

Stokes, R., & Faris, D. D. (1983). *Fitness Everyone.* Winston-Salem, NC: Hunter.

Stokes, R., Moore, A. C., & Moore, C. (1986). *Fitness: The New Wave.* 2d ed. Winston-Salem, NC: Hunter.

Sweetgall, R., & Dignam, J. (1986). *The Walker's Journal.* Newark, DE: Creative Walking.

Sweetgall, R., Rippe, J., & Katch, F. (1985). *Rockport's Fitness Walking.* New York: Putnam.

Terry, J. W., Johnson, D. J., & Erickson, C. R. (1984). *Physical Activity for All Ages: Concepts of High-Level Wellness.* 2d ed. Dubuque, IA: Kendall/Hunt.

Thaxton, N. A. (1988). *Pathways to Fitness: Foundations, Motivation, Applications.* New York: Harper & Row.

Tufts University Diet and Nutrition Letter. (June 1992). *Fifty Simple Ways to Improve Your Diet* (Vol. 10, No. 4). Park Place, NY.

Tufts University Diet and Nutrition Letter. (July 1992). *Government Gives New Shape to Eating Right* (Vol. 10, No. 5). Park Place, NY.

Turner, L. W., Sizer, F. S., Whitney, E. N., & Wilks, B. B. (1992). *Life Choices: Health Concepts and Strategies.* 2d ed. St. Paul: West.

U.S. Department of Agriculture, U.S. Department of Health and Human Resources. (1990). *Nutrition and Your Health: Dietary Guidelines for Americans.* 3d ed. Washington, DC: Government Printing Office.

Van Itallie, T. B., & Kral, J. G. (August 28, 1981). The Dilemma of Morbid Obesity. *Journal of the American Medical Association,* 246, 999–1003.

Vitale, F. (1973). *Individualized Fitness Programs.* Englewood Cliffs, NJ: Prentice-Hall.

Walcott, G., Coleman, R., MacVeigh, M., Ross, J., Gurry, M., Ward, A., Kline, G., & Rippe, J. (1986). Heart Rate and $\dot{V}O_2$ max Response to Weighted Walking. *Medicine and Science in Sports and Exercise,* 18, S28.

Walking for Fitness, a Round Table. (October 1986). *The Physician and Sportsmedicine,* 14(10), 145–149.

Ward, A., Wilkie, S., O'Hanley, S., Trask, C., Kallmes, D., Kleinerman, J., Crawford, B., Freedson, P., & Rippe, J. (1987). Estimation of $\dot{V}O_2$ max in Overweight Females. *Medicine and Science in Sports and Exercise,* 19, 528.

Weinberg, R., Caldwell, P., Cornelius, W., Jackson, A., & Smith, J. (1982). *Health Related Fitness: Theory and Practice.* Topeka, KS: Jostens.

Wilkie, S., O'Hanley, S., Ward, A., Zwiren, L., Freedson, P., Crawford, B., Kleinerman, J., & Rippe, J. (1987). Estimation of $\dot{V}O_2$ max from a One-Mile Walk Test Using Recovery Heart Rate. *Medicine and Science in Sports and Exercise,* 19, 528.

Williams, M. H. (1985). *Lifetime Physical Fitness: A Personal Choice.* Dubuque, IA: Wm. C. Brown.

Wilmore, J. H., & Costill, D. L. (1988). *Training for Sport and Activity: The Physiological Basis of the Conditioning Process.* 3d ed. Dubuque, IA: Wm. C. Brown.

Yanker, G. (1983). *The Complete Book of Exercisewalking.* Chicago: Contemporary.

Yanker, G. (1985). *Gary Yanker's Walking Workouts.* New York: Warner.

Zwiren, L. D., Freedson, P. S., Ward, A., Wilkie, S., & Rippe, J. (1987). Prediction of $\dot{V}O_2$ max: Comparison of 5 Submaximal Tests. *Medicine and Science in Sports and Exercise,* 19, 564.

Index